THE DIET THA⌐ WORKS

By Kevin G. Myles

Table of Contents

A special thank you to my family and all of my wonderful friends and clients!

Kevin

FORWARD

My Fitness Evolution
by Elaine Goodlad
(Pro Figure Champion and Top Fitness Model)

Many times when people see someone who is fit and healthy, they make the mistake of assuming that it came easily for that person or that they must have always been this way. The truth is that many of today's fittest people started out with a lot of obstacles and were able to improve their appearance simply because they wanted to.

There was a time in my life when things were not going very well. Because of certain emotional situations I went through, I developed low self-esteem and was quite depressed.

To combat my depression, I began to overeat because food was always a source of comfort and good feelings when I was growing up. Pretty soon I had gained a ton of weight and my depression grew worse. I started forcing myself to throw up after binging on food as a way to find the comfort that I desperately needed while trying to control my weight. My life had gotten way out of hand and I felt like I had no control.

My cousin Betty saw I was not doing well. She convinced me to come to the gym with her to feel better and find a more constructive way of controlling my weight. That was my first introduction to the gym and weight training, just about 20 years ago.

Ultimately, I started working out with a friend of mine who taught me a lot about training hard, eating right, and the benefits of living a fitness lifestyle. I began to re-learn how to value myself as I put my energy into this new, positive fitness lifestyle. Through his encouragement, I again became able to see my own value and was able to adopt much more positive behavior. Sometimes it takes someone else to help you see the good things in yourself. That was about 18 years ago. We eventually fell in love and were married. We still train together and we also work together and are best friends.

I still struggle with food and wanting to throw up from time to time but those times are rare and I am in control. Living a fit lifestyle has given me confidence and has changed my self-image. Every trip to the gym, every cardio session, every meal, is a challenge with rewards that I see every day. Eating well is very easy to do and the odd cheat day is part of the program so it's not a failure. Outside of normal cravings when dieting, I never have the urge to gorge myself. My comfort comes now from feeling healthy, looking good, and knowing I have worked hard for all I have. Inspiring others to look after themselves and improve their self-worth gives purpose to all the work and sacrifice required to be an athlete and model. I feel that God gave me those struggles and challenges so I could eventually inspire others and serving him is my life's purpose. That is my reason for competing, modeling, and being here for those that he sends my way. As you continue your fitness journey, I hope I can be a source of inspiration to you because if I can do it, you can as well.

God Bless

Elaine Goodlad

www.elainefit.com
www.bodysport.com

Becoming a Diamond: Investing in Yourself Through Fitness.

In this day and age, you'd have to be from Mars not to know that diamonds are precious and valuable. Yet their value only came about over great periods of time and involved quite a bit of change. The end product is merely the result of those changes and the external forces and pressures that brought them about. A great physique, your dream physique, is also an end product. It will come from a combination of planned changes that take place over time. But like someone who has never heard of a diamond, if you have never had or seen this dream physique of yours, it's hard to appreciate the value it will have or even believe in the possibility of its existence. Why should you put your time, effort, and energy into attaining something if you don't know its true value, or if you're not sure you can ever have it? The inability to see the value of practicing a fitness lifestyle, or to believe we can achieve the desired results, are the two biggest factors that prevent us from reaching our fitness goals. It is within our minds and our hearts that we develop the ability to "become a diamond". All it takes is a little self-investment.

We all make investments into something or someone. We invest in our cars, children, spouse, careers, friends, homes, etc. These investments can involve time, money, patience, hope, work, or a number of other things. Yet, other than our school years, we don't always find the time to invest in ourselves. It is easy for us to see the value and reward of external investment, but often we don't put the same level of importance into improving ourselves. What we need to understand is that by investing in ourselves, we are investing in everything and everyone around us at the same time. By increasing our own value and ability, we are able to give more and do more for others. Every self-investment we make can create a better situation for those we come in contact with. By improving ourselves, we increase our value to others. One of the best ways to self-invest is by adopting a fitness lifestyle.

One of the things that I have learned from my recent seminars is that just having the right information is not always enough. Basically there are two types of people that I tend to work with. One group consists of people who have been trying to make improvements but for some reason are not getting the results they desire. I have spent most of my fitness life learning and teaching the information to help this group of people become successful. Most recently my focus has been on a second group. This is the group that would like to be in better shape, but have not been able to get themselves to adopt a fitness lifestyle. Unfortunately, this is an even larger group with greater health concerns. I now dedicate the opening segment of my seminars to addressing the people in this group. It is an even greater challenge because it ultimately doesn't depend upon what information I can give someone, but whether or not they choose to utilize the information. The message I try to deliver to them is really quite simple. When it comes to fitness, often it is not so much what you do or how you do it as it is finding a reason why you should. Once you find the "Why" you will much more easily discover the "How".

Everywhere we turn our reality is invaded by some aspect of the fitness crusade. Whether it's a new diet, special weight-loss potion, magic energy pill, 2-for-1 gym ad, or the latest 3-minute total body workout apparatus, our senses are being constantly bombarded until we become almost immune to the information. We get to the point where we can't tell the good from the bad and for the most part don't care. Then, in some moment of out-of-shape desperation, we pump ourselves up and dive into the fitness ocean, heedless of sharks, freezing temperatures, or the fact that we can't swim a lick. It's no wonder that we soon wind up in over our heads, exhausted, and just wishing to get back to the shores of a normal life. We convince ourselves that some things just weren't meant to be and probably aren't worth the effort anyway. It's not our bodies that have failed us, but our minds and our spirits that have been let down. Before we can achieve physical success, we must understand mentally and emotionally how valuable and capable we truly are.

In order to reach your fitness goals, you have to believe and know that you will reach them, no matter what. There cannot be any doubt in your mind or you will not commit yourself to making the necessary changes. I have seen people accomplish amazing things with time, effort, and a little knowledge. You have the power to change your life by investing in your health through fitness. Becoming fit will create more energy, longevity, greater self-esteem, increased strength and stamina, and generally improve your outlook on life. A great percentage of the people today who enjoy health and fitness did not start out that way. They transformed themselves into their physical ideals and there is absolutely no reason that you can't do the same. The biggest first step is throwing away your doubts and apprehensions. Those are the things that keep you from committing because you are not sure if your efforts will be properly rewarded. I promise you that not only will the results you get be worth your efforts, but that you will receive wonderful rewards that go beyond outward physical improvement. Much greater than the visual rewards will be the way your new fitness lifestyle brings out and highlights all of the positive things about you and allows them to direct your life. You will develop a new and improved self image that comes with a more positive outlook and the confidence that you can overcome any challenge that life has to offer. These are capabilities that we all have, but sometimes need help bringing out. Following a fitness lifestyle can help you unleash potential you never knew you possessed. There is not a person I know who has adopted this lifestyle that would tell you anything different.

The other big obstacle also has to do with self worth. It is a question that stems from our own natural insecurities. In regards to adopting a fitness lifestyle, all too many people worry not so much is "it" worth it but are "they" worth it. A lot of people seem to lack a personal sense of self importance and don't feel that they are worth putting the time, effort, and energy into. Nothing can be further from the truth. Even if you don't see it or feel it, your value to yourself and the world around you is so great that it is impossible to measure. Small changes in your life and a new focus can bring out qualities in you that you weren't even aware of. All it takes is a little self-investment to begin unlocking the rest of your potential and put you in a position where your greatest attributes can easily be seen. Confidence, self-esteem, helpfulness, patience, knowledge, compassion, determination and many other characteristics which you may not even know you posses are ready to rush to the forefront of your life with just a little encouragement. It may seem amazing to you that just being more fit and healthy can cause all this to take place, but once you start down the path of fitness you will begin to see and feel many great changes taking place. The greatest thing is that well before you reach your final goal, you will know that a positive transformation is taking place.

I can tell you of a time personally when my greatest wish as I walked down the street was that I could become invisible. Such was the level of my self-image at the time that for all the things that I was capable of athletically and academically, this was truly my wish. If I were invisible, no one would be able to see any of my self-perceived flaws, right? From that base, I developed into a person who looks forward to public speaking and meeting new people. It's certainly not because I now feel flawless, but because I understand that it's OK not to be, and that our flaws make us unique and special. I also discovered that our strengths are much greater than our weaknesses once we develop the ability to see them. My involvement with fitness taught me these things and much more. The numerous values of implementing a fitness lifestyle that many people discover by accident are now goals to be pursued with purpose.

So now it's up to you to go out there and live your fitness life. Take up walking, join a gym, play basketball, start swimming, become a runner, lift weights, practice yoga, study martial arts, practice cardio kickboxing, eat more healthy, get a physical, stop smoking, cut down on drinking, be more positive, love yourself, renew your faith, and enjoy your life. Whatever you choose to do will be worth it because you are worth it. You will create greater health and therefore greater opportunities for yourself and your life. You will discover powers that you never knew you had and they will be to the benefit of everyone around you. Your already incredible value will become much easier to see all because of a little self-investment through fitness. And this specialness will never go away, but only increase in value with time, both to yourself and to others. Just like a diamond!

THE DIET THAT WORKS©

CHAPTER 1

What you need to know about losing weight

With very few exceptions, most people will go through a period of time when they will need or want to lose weight. For some it might be just a few pounds. For others, it could be quite a bit more. Some people will have little problem being successful while others will only become more frustrated as they just don't seem to be able to get the results they want. Well, I'm here to let you know that not only can you achieve the results you seek, but also to tell you how. There are reasons why some people have success and others do not. In over 30-years of being involved in the fitness industry I have seen all levels and variations of hopes and dreams become either dashed or fulfilled. I have seen and heard countless stories and accounts of what has and has not worked. I have watched people get rich on misinformation and deceit, promoting nutrition programs and diets that weren't fit for human consumption while preying on the hopeful enthusiasm of the naive. I always knew there was a better way. The time has come for someone to show it to you.

You should probably know that I never really intended to do a book on weight-loss or diet. This has all come about due to two things; my ability to learn and my desire to help. I became involved in exercise and fitness out of pure enjoyment. I remember getting up in the morning with my sister and working out with Jack and Elaine Lalane in the family living room. Jack was so full of energy, life, and enthusiasm that even my six-year old mind could grasp the importance of what he was trying to say beyond simply learning how to do jumping jacks. Being fit was something that I was fortunate enough to discover early. And when injuries and

9

circumstances caused me to lose the level of fitness I had once possessed, I knew from having been there how important it was to recapture.

Even at the stages in my life where I was most fit, I never considered that this made me better than anyone, only more fortunate. I noticed that certain things that I had once taken for granted would have been considered outright blessings by others. So I always made it a point to be as helpful as possible whenever I was fortunate enough to have that opportunity. I started out by answering a few questions here and there. Over time this evolved into designing workout and nutrition plans for friends and acquaintances. I even started doing free personal training at my college weight room where I worked part time. As I continued to learn more and more, my answers became longer and longer to the point where I knew that simply telling someone part of the story was not really helping them. I started to write down the basic information that seemed to be desired by everyone and made it available as handouts when I started working in a health food store once I finished college. As the information became more and more elaborate and involved, I knew that ultimately I would have to sit down and specifically address a number of topics.

I will tell you right now that I am not a doctor or dietician. Nor will I be prescribing to you or attempting to cure or improve upon any disease that you might have. Without boring you with details I will tell you that I have coached and/or advised a number of high level athletes as well as absolute beginners. I have completed numerous certification courses and have been doing personal training and nutritional consultations for 30 years. I have spent 15 years managing health food stores, gyms, exercise equipment stores, and involving myself in health and fitness by interacting with hundreds of people on a number of different levels. I have given seminars on weight-loss and nutrition at corporate facilities and have written for the most popular websites and magazines in the fitness industry. I have successfully counseled more people than I can count on matters involving exercise, nutrition, and weight management. None of this really matters. The only thing that matters is whether or not I can help you. I believe that I can. I challenge you to trust me and believe in yourself and your ability to make the changes you desire.

The need for change: Before we go any further, there is one thing that you must understand and accept. **In order to get the results you want, you must be willing to make some changes. It doesn't matter if I give you the greatest information in the world, if you continue to do exactly what you have been doing all of your life, you will achieve exactly the same results you have had all of your life**. Now, before you become concerned, we might be talking about some very small changes. There may just be one or two things you need to do a little differently in order to get you on your way. If a lot of changes are required of you, rest assured that they will not be so difficult that you can't make them and that they will be for your own benefit. Some of this will be re-learning proper behavior and incorporating better habits. Some of it will be learning and implementing information that you simply weren't aware of. But rest assured, if no changes were required then you would already be exactly where you want to be. But I know you can do everything you need to do to make things happen for yourself.

This is for you: It is very important for you to understand that this is something you should be doing for yourself simply because you want to. No one, not a parent or spouse or co-worker or "mainstream society" can or should force you into making changes that you do not want to make. If you draw energy or inspiration from outside sources, people, or influences, that is fine. Just as long as the ultimate reason you are attempting to accomplish this or any other task is because you believe it is important and valuable and should be done. It is this belief that will fuel your desire even if everyone else around you disappears.

Develop a sense of worth: Do you really have any idea how special and unique and valuable you are? Do you understand your own worth? Sometimes we get the proper feedback through interactions with others to help us know this, but most of the time, we don't. I am here to tell you that you are as important and meaningful as anyone who has ever lived and you deserve every good thing you could possibly have. A lot of times, when we don't perceive ourselves as perfect, we don't perceive our proper value either. I've got news for you, all of those "perfect people" out there aren't perfect either. You have just as much right to happiness and fulfillment as anyone. The reason I say this to you is that oftentimes people think that once they accomplish a certain goal, a lot of things will get better because then they will be more deserving. What I want you to understand and believe is that being leaner, or smarter, or richer, or prettier, or whatever, will not make you more special. **You already are that special!** Accomplishing goals just allows us to see ourselves in a more positive light and appreciate our own specialness all the more. Don't wait to start feeling good about yourself and how special you are. You should start believing right this very moment how important you are and how any amount of time and effort it takes to bring this part of yourself more to the front is time and effort well spent because you are tremendously valuable and truly worth it!

The Power of Belief: Of all the people I have ever coached you can separate the ones who've achieved and maintained success from the ones who didn't by one thing. **In order to be successful, you have to believe that you will be. Your power to control your own destiny when it comes to losing weight is absolute. You are the one who will make it happen and nothing or no one can stop you.** By believing in yourself and your ultimate success, you will be better able to focus on the tasks that are necessary for you to achieve your goals. The information I will give you will teach you everything you need to know to maximize your look. You just have to believe in your ability to put forth the necessary effort and implement the proper changes to make your dreams a reality. Yes, there are things beyond our control. I cannot make you taller, or younger, or fly like a bird. But I can give you all the information you will need to reach your goals. You just have to believe this is something that can and will happen for you and that this time it's your turn to be successful.

Why people are overweight: One of the reasons that so many people in the world have trouble keeping and maintaining a proper bodyweight is simply genetics or more specifically, natural selection. Our ancestors did not have the luxury of having food readily available to them. Hunting and scavenging for food was a survival necessity. Often they would have to go days with little or nothing to eat. In order to survive, they had to become very efficient at storing food. Well, the body's way of storing food is through producing fat. It is an efficient source of energy and insulation against the cold. The people who survived long enough to produce and raise offspring had the most efficient fat storing metabolisms. To this day, our bodies still contain survival mechanisms that cause us to store consumed excess fat, carbohydrates, and protein as adipose tissue. And since the advances of civilization have led to most of us living in a society that no longer balances our energy expenditures with our caloric intake, we have a tendency to put on unwanted weight if we are not careful. There are some specific metabolic and physiological factors involved that I will get into later but the important thing for you to know is this; you are overweight simply because that's how your body was designed to work. It is not because you are a bad person or a weak person or that you don't have enough will power or determination. You simply have a very calorically efficient metabolism.   This is also truer for some than for others. The good news is, there are ways around this and I will teach them to you.

Alleviating the Guilt and Accepting the Responsibility: As important as it is to understand how the body works physiologically, it is even more important to understand that everyone is unique, not just physically, but also mentally, intellectually, and emotionally. That is why no one program can be perfect for everyone. The good thing about what I will teach you is that it is not "just one program" but a way of adapting the principles and rules of effective weight-loss to formulate your own individual program. We have all seen the person who can seemingly eat anything and everything and never gain a pound. In contrast to that, others of us can just look at food and our weight increases. Wherever you happen to fall on the "ease of gaining weight" continuum, obviously some have it easier than others. Just as obviously, there is no reason for you to feel guilty about not being as lean as someone metabolically more fortunate than you. The frustration of having a more difficult road can lead to a defeatist attitude and the incorporation of bad habits that keep you from improving. That is why there is something you must do right now. You must absolve yourself of all guilt you might feel about being overweight. Chances are the initial reasons for this happening were out of your control because you didn't fully understand what was going on. Don't beat yourself up for not being where you would like to be. This will only make you question whether you deserve for things to be different which shouldn't even be a consideration. You should be fully and exactly where you would like to be. By the same token you must also <u>right now</u> accept responsibility for what happens from here on. There is a cause and effect relationship between what you do, how you eat, and how you look. Knowing this gives you the ability to effectively control and change yourself. This is the type of power you have always had but maybe you didn't know it. You are totally in control of how you will ultimately look and it is a great power to posses, and a great feeling to have when you are utilizing that power.

Getting Started: What is a Diet?

Before we go any further, let's first make sure you know what a diet is. The word diet has become synonymous with periods of self imposed deprivation and borderline starvation. It has come to represent a state of mind and action that promotes temporary changes that can only lead to failure.   Simply put, a diet is the sum total of what we eat and drink everyday. And depending upon what that consists of and what your goals are, your diet can be either good or bad. A diet is not something to go on and off. Instead it should be thought of as a permanent eating lifestyle or philosophy that, with periodic adjustments, will allow you to have control over how you feel, how you look, and to a large degree, how healthy you are. The way we eat has an effect on us physically and by understanding that, we can control those effects if we desire.

Awareness vs. Denial: A lot of what you will accomplish and how rapidly will be determined by whether you are existing in a state of awareness or living in denial in terms of your current eating habits. Before you can fix something, you need to know where and how it is broken. Good or bad, we as humans are blessed with the incredible ability to simply ignore the obvious even when it's right in front of us and/or a part of our daily lives. Subconsciously we know when we are practicing eating habits that are undesirable but we can become very practiced at blocking them out. A very important step in your ultimately becoming successful is developing absolute awareness of everything you are doing as it relates to your nutritional program. This doesn't mean that you have to eat perfectly or that you can never have any fun foods like pizza or ice cream and cake. What it means is that you must be conscious and aware of everything that you are consuming. No more living in denial and I mean starting right now. The reason for this is simple. The things that you do consciously you can ultimately control. It is the things that you do un-consciously or without thinking that can create problems for you, at least until you develop a better set of habits.

The Importance of Structure: Just about every difficult accomplishment can be made noticeably easier with a good plan and every good plan involves structure. If you were trying to increase your knowledge by going to college and getting a degree, you wouldn't start by randomly walking around campus, sticking your head into a few classrooms and hoping to learn the information you needed. You would have a very specific course schedule designed to make sure you efficiently covered all the required areas. In order to have maximum productivity in the work place, everyone has a specific task and schedule and is required to perform according to some overall plan or goal. The same must be true for your nutrition program if you desire to make it work in your favor. You cannot expect to randomly put things into your mouth at any given time of the day without any regards to what your actual needs might be and no way to recall how much you did or didn't have. There needs to be a structured program with specific goals, guidelines, and timeframes. This will give you the opportunity to plan, monitor, control, and adjust your intake. This ability will be a key factor in allowing you to determine what is and isn't working for you and have the chance to do something about it. By adding structure to your eating habits you eliminate the powerlessness that has existed in your life because even when you are not eating "perfectly", you will have the ability to see what is actually going on and the power to change and modify it. When you combine the power and ability to monitor and change with the responsibility of self-determination, you will be on your way to achieving success.

Starting now, write down everything you eat and drink along with the times. This is one of the first things I have my clients do. I usually have them start with the prior two days so that they can't alter their habits and I have them keep track for one week. Then I am able to analyze their diet and see where and how they need to make changes. One of the biggest discoveries I've made with this is how much more conscious my clients become of what they are doing by having to write it down. It creates not only a sense of awareness but also a sense of accountability because they have to face that written record of their choices and habits, something that little thing called denial didn't require them to do. So, it is imperative, starting right now that you write down everything you eat and drink. In fact, start from two days ago (and don't pretend that you can't remember because I know you can). This will give you three-days of info and you'll have enough to work with in order to start taking control of your progress. We are not looking for good or bad, we just need to see what your body is used to and we need to start developing your awareness. Don't plan on stopping any time soon. I would suggest using a spiral notebook, and no matter what, make sure you write everything down. For now don't worry about calories or grams or amounts, we simply want times and substances. That little spiral notebook will be a tremendous tool for you in helping to put you in the position of power and control.

Analyzing Your Info. So, how do you make the information you have in your notebook work for you? The biggest benefit of having awareness is the opportunities you now have to better control the situation. Take a look at the food and drink recordings in your log book. The first things that will stand out are the items that you know were not exactly conducive to weight-loss. Hey, that's OK, you don't need to eat "perfectly" in order to be fit, lean, and healthy. We are just trying to make you take account of your own habits and actions. It's not that you will never have those foods again, it's just that you need to plan when to have them, be aware of when you are having them and their effect on you, and not have them to the degree that they will keep you from reaching your goals. By having them written down in front of you, you can begin to see where and when you need to cut down. One thing I have noticed with the people I coach is that just the reality of having to write down everything you eat leads to a noticeable decrease in the consumption of the less than ideal foods. This is because you will no longer be operating in a state of denial and you are beginning to take control. Congratulations when this happens to you. It is a very important step.

The other things you need to look at are; how often you are eating, how long you go between meals, what times of the day you are eating, and what types of foods and drinks you are consuming. Each one of these factors has a specific effect upon your progress and will be addressed in order to maximize your results. For now, your focus should be on learning as much as you can about your own habits in order to take conscious control of your actions and ultimately, your results.

Taking a Lifestyle Approach. As you begin to acquire and analyze information, there is something I would like to emphasis to you. **Although it is possible to make rapid changes and lose weight quickly, it is not the speed of the weight-loss you should be concerned with as much as the permanence of the weight-loss.** It really doesn't make sense to approach your diet in a way that leads only to temporary changes. I am sure many of us have lost weight through effort and sacrifice, only to have it return all too soon. These types of programs make for great advertising copy, **"Lose Weight Now Without Diet or Exercise!"** But the sad reality is that they seldom work with any permanence other than to make someone else rich off of your desire to improve. Don't get me wrong, I have nothing against riches, I just happen to think that truth and health are more important. That is why you need to understand that you should never do anything detrimental to your health in order to achieve a cosmetic effect. No pills, potions, or radical programs done at the expense of your well being will give you results any better than if you simply learn more about how your body works and implement certain changes in your nutritional habits and lifestyle. **There is no secret or easy way! But there is an easier, more effective approach if you accept it!** That is by making a commitment to your own health and happiness to make the changes in your lifestyle that support the results you desire to have. Of course it takes time to change habits and philosophies and it will be an ongoing project. But the benefits of these changes will enhance your life far beyond any changes you see on the scale. The things that I'll have you do will cause you to lose unwanted weight, but the principles you incorporate as part of a lifestyle change will insure that you never have to deal with a weight problem again. Knowledge is power and that is the one gift I can give to you, the knowledge to improve and control your look. But you are the one that has to actually open this gift and start to utilize it. Once you do, the changes on the scale, as great as they may be, will pale in comparison to the changes in your eyes and in your smile.

Proper Eating Frequency: Getting back to your food log, one of the key things you should always be aware of is how often you are eating. If you are only eating once or twice a day you will effectively be slowing down your metabolism and making it more difficult to get lean. Always remember that your body is geared primarily for survival and this is manifested as energy conservation and storage. When you go a long period of time without eating it's almost as if your body interprets this by saying "Oh no, we must be starving!" and proceeds to start trying to conserve energy by slowing down your metabolic rate. Then, when you eat again your body is still in survival mode and does its best to store as much reserve energy as possible. In other words, the practice of eating meals few and far between will make it harder for you to burn calories and easier for you to store them. This is exactly the opposite of what you want. **By eating more frequently throughout the day, your metabolism will remain active and you will be burning more calories without your body feeling the need to activate survival mechanisms.** Also, eating more frequently will help maintain a more constant blood sugar level. This will cause less cravings and hunger and therefore reduce the likelihood of you not being in control of your intake. Ideally, you want to work up to consuming 5-6 smaller or moderate meals a day as opposed to 2-3 large ones. Many of the competitors I coach eat a minimum of six times a day and they are the leanest people you will ever meet. It's all about training your body to be metabolically efficient. This is the state where you have plenty of energy and an active metabolism that utilizes the nourishment which is provided with minimal fat storage.

If you are currently eating only 1-3 meals a day, you don't want to jump up to 5-6. That would be too much of a shock for your system. You always want to make changes gradually to give yourself adequate time to adjust. Remember, we are talking about lifestyle changes. It is also a change to prepare five meals a day when you were previously only concerned with a couple. Try adding one extra meal a day at the rate of every 1-2 weeks. This will give you the time you need to adjust both physically and mentally. As your body gets accustomed to eating more frequently, your metabolic rate should begin to increase. Initially you may find that it helps to utilize the clock and try to eat around the same time everyday. It will take a little getting used to and I caution you not to force feed yourself but do give yourself those extra feedings you will need to kick start your metabolism. If you are not feeling hungry and can go all day on only a couple of meals, that's a good sign that your metabolism is sluggish. Once you start eating more often, you won't have to look at the clock to know when it's time to eat, your body will tell you as you will get hungry a lot more frequently. You will quickly go from saying. "Man it's time to eat again?" to saying "I can't believe I'm hungry again, when is it time to eat?" Once you get to the later point that is a sign that your metabolism is starting to work the way you need it to. This is a very important step and it means you are heading in the right direction.

Choosing Foods and Making Meals: Another thing that is vitally important to look at is how each meal is structured. This is probably one of the most confusing and debated aspects of nutrition. There are entire diets based solely on this content. The trick is, how do you know which is best for you? Well, the answer is easy, you let your body tell you.

There are basic nutrients that you need from the standpoint of having and maintaining ideal health. Known as the six elements of food they are; protein, carbohydrates, fats, vitamins, minerals, and water. I could write an entire article on each of these and their functions but for the sake of this book we're going to focus on the information you need for your weight-loss program. When putting together your diet or analyzing your food log a big concern should be, **"Are the foods you're consuming actually nourishing your body?"** Do they have nutritional value? On the whole, as a society we consume: too much sugar, too much fat, too great a percentage of the wrong type of fats, too much sodium, not enough vitamins, minerals, and antioxidants, and for most people with a weight problem a diet that has too high a percentage of carbohydrates vs. protein. This can leave quite a few things to fix but there is a simple way to do this that is very effective and that I promise won't overwhelm you.

Notice that one thing I didn't say is that we are consuming too many calories. A lot of times this isn't the problem as much as consuming the wrong types of calories at the wrong times of day. Many people can actually eat more than they do. It's just a matter of making better choices and increasing your activity level. **The best way to insure you are eating properly is to focus on what you should be having, not on what you shouldn't be having**.

CHAPTER 2

Putting Your Meals Together

Step 1 –Make sure each meal contains protein: The word protein literally means, "Of first importance" and that is the first and most important step you should take in your meal preparation. **Virtually every meal you consume (with a few exceptions for athletes from a performance or recovery standpoint) should contain protein.** There are ongoing debates among various health care professionals, trainers, nutritionists, and athletes about how much protein you actually need to consume. When in doubt, always let health and logic be your guide. The fact of the matter is you need a certain amount of calories throughout the day. These calories must come from somewhere. If you are trying to lose fat, you will most likely need to consume only a healthy amount of fats and a controlled amount of carbohydrates. That leaves you to get the rest of your calories from protein.

The body can only digest and assimilate so much protein (or any type of food) at one time. At the same time, the body can't store protein the way it does fat and carbohydrates so you need to take it in periodically throughout the day. This is another reason why dividing your daily food intake up into smaller, more manageable portions is an effective approach. Among people in the fitness community the daily protein recommendation will range anywhere from a minimum of a gram of protein per kilogram (2.2 pounds) of body weight to a gram of protein (or more) per pound of body weight. Without getting into the heated debate, I will tell you what I feel is best for you.

It would be almost impossible for you to get enough of the right kind of calories throughout the day without consuming at least a gram of protein per pound of your target body weight. Notice I said target weight. What I mean by this is, if you weigh 250 and your goal is to reach 175, then that is your target body weight and you should be consuming about 175 grams of protein a day as a starting point. Now let's say you're consuming 150 grams of protein a day. Since protein has 4 calories per gram, that is 600 calories. That's really not a whole lot for an entire day. The rest of your calories will come from either carbohydrates, which also has 4 calories per gram, or fat which has 9 calories per gram. And since you are trying to get a better handle on your fat and carbohydrate intakes, the more protein you consume, the less carbohydrates and fats you will need to consume to make up the balance of your caloric intake. (Alcohol has about 7 calories per gram but we are not including alcohol as a part of your normal diet).

So what's the best way to get the proper amount? Listen to your body. You know better than anyone how much food it takes to satisfy your hunger. Initially, we don't want to alter the amount of your intake, we simply want to change the makeup of your intake. By eating cleaner and healthier, you will be able to lower your caloric intake without feeling hungry or deprived. In fact, you actually may be eating more food than normal due to greater consistency in maintaining meal frequency, but because of food selection, the amount of calories you consume will be less and this will start the desired changes in your body composition. The first step to getting the ideal meal balance is making sure each meal contains an adequate amount of protein. I usually recommend a minimum of 20-25 grams of protein per meal for my female clients and 35-40 grams per meal for my male clients. Please utilize the food logs towards the end of this book to get the nutritional contents of a variety of foods. Just to give you a quick example, one 94% lean ground beef patty would be 25 grams of protein, and one 3.5 ounce chicken breast would be 36 grams of protein. Definitely not more than you are capable of eating. The key is that every meal should contain a protein source.

Step 2-Use your energy needs to determine your carbohydrate intake: Carbohydrate foods are getting such a bad rap in the media right now that it's almost laughable. The popularity of low-carb diets has more to do with marketing and lack of knowledge than it does with healthy weight-loss or good nutrition. You do not need to eliminate carbohydrates from your diet in order to effectively lose weight. In fact, one of the big problems with losing weight on a low-carb diet is that it is some of the easiest weight to gain back. Carbohydrate foods contain vital vitamins, minerals, fiber, antioxidants, and trace elements that are essential to good health. They are also the body's most efficient energy source. While it is true that processed carbohydrates and simple sugars can be quite unhealthy and contribute greatly to unwanted weight-gain and obesity, complex carbohydrates such as whole grains, beans, legumes, vegetables, and fruits are quite healthy and should never be completely removed from the diet. Your nutrition program should be about more than achieving a cosmetic effect. It should be about becoming fit and healthy with an abundance of energy and vitality. Having a lean and attractive physique is simply a wonderful side effect of taking a lifestyle approach to health, fitness, and nutrition.

That being said, one of the best ways to control your body composition is through manipulation (not elimination) of your carb intake. Since your protein intake will remain relatively constant throughout the day and from meal-to-meal, and your fat intake should be kept to a healthy minimum, it is your carbohydrate intake that you should use to fine tune your diet. It's not just enough to evenly divide your meals and/or calories up throughout the day in terms of amount. There are times of the day when you will be expending more energy than normal and times when you will be using less. At each meal, you should ask yourself, "What will I be doing over the next 3-4 hours?" Obviously if you are going to be taking a nap or sitting and watching television you won't need as much energy as you would if you were going to be mowing the lawn or heading to the gym for a workout. Having a foresighted approach to your energy needs will allow you to fine-tune your carbohydrate intake so that you can insure that you have enough energy for your periods of greater activity, but you don't over consume before your periods of inactivity. Obviously plans change as things come up unexpectedly but taking this type of approach to your meal planning is very effective and gives you a lot of control over your diet.

Unlike with protein, every meal you have should not contain carbs or at least complex carbs. But there are times even while "dieting" when you can and should have carbohydrates in terms of maximum health, energy, and weight maintenance. Usually for people who are on a weight-loss program I recommend that the last meal of the day contain no complex carbs and consist of only protein and fibrous carbs like vegetables or a salad and some healthy fats. This will help insure that your blood sugar is not elevated when you sleep and your body will be more capable of releasing its own natural hormones like growth hormone which has great fat burning capabilities. Effective growth hormone release is greatly influenced by nutrition and having a relatively empty stomach is ideal. Not eating within the last 1-2 hours before bedtime and not having any complex carbohydrate foods for at least 4-5 hours before bedtime has worked very well for a number of people I have coached. (For the record, when I mention fibrous carbohydrates I am referring to insoluble fiber carbs like vegetables which really don't add an appreciable amount of calories when you eat them as they consist primarily of non-digestible fiber and water. Soluble fiber carbohydrates like oat bran, rolled oats, and apple fiber do contribute calories and are complex carbohydrates. Research has shown that this type of fiber is great for helping to lower cholesterol levels.)

So what's a quick way to know if you're putting the right amount of carbs on your plate? Of the meals in which you will eat complex carbs you will pretty much be eating anywhere from the same amount of carbs as protein up to twice as much carbs as protein based upon how much energy you will need. Yes, this can always be adjusted but it is a good basic starting point that won't require much effort on your part and will instantly put you in control over your program. To illustrate what this would look like, lets say you're a female who is eating 25 grams of protein per meal. You have worked your way up to four meals a day with the goal of reaching five. Your fourth or last meal will only contain protein and fibrous carbs. That leaves three other meals. Since the early part of your day will be pretty sedentary followed by a 30-minute walk on the treadmill after work, you know that your energy needs will be minimal after the first two meals and greater after meal three.

Under these circumstances you would break down your daily diet as follows:

Meal 1: Protein 25 grams, Complex Carbs-25 grams, Fibrous Carbs
Meal 2: Protein 25 grams, Complex Carbs-25 grams, Fibrous Carbs
Meal 3: Protein 25 grams, Complex Carbs-50 grams, Fibrous Carbs
Meal 4: Protein 25 grams, Complex Carbs-0 grams, Fibrous Carbs

Pretty simple and very individual. All you have to do is choose your sources of protein and carbs then prepare and consume your meals. If hunger gets to be a problem, remember that we are trying to get you to at least five meals anyway. Meal 5 would then look like Meal 4 and your 4th meal would have 25 grams of protein, 0-50 grams of complex carbs depending on your goals and energy needs and as much fibrous carbs as you would like. By the way, if the above example seems like a lot of food, as written it is only 800 calories which is way too few! Remember, those protein suggestions are minimum amounts and some of your caloric intake will come from healthy fats. Once you have your diet structured in this manner it will be quite easy to adjust it based upon how you respond. You will have the ability to control and fine tune your eating program based upon energy needs, hunger, weight changes, and daily schedule. It will take you only a couple of weeks to know how your body will respond and design the perfect program for yourself. Once you have this ability, you will be able to lose as much as you need to lose simply by making minor changes within a couple of meals and you will never lose this ability!

If it sounds too good to be true, trust me, it really isn't. There are, however, some other tips and facts that I will tell you to make this program more effective than just playing with your caloric control through structured food selection and macronutrient percentages. (Fancy words for what we just did). However, first I will give you an example of just how well this works.

Personal Experience: The first time I ever found myself in need of losing weight was before my first bodybuilding competition. Being a lifetime drug-free athlete, it had been quite a struggle for me to put on an appreciable amount of muscle size that I would need to be competitive. After years of training and eating as many calories a day as I could, (Including using a lot of weight-gain drinks) I discovered that although I had gained size, too much of the weight I put on had been fat and I would now need to lose it for my competition which was in three months. If you know anything about bodybuilding then you know that the accepted standards for competition leanness are quite extreme. Having little information to work with (I thought I had a lot of good sources but what I didn't know about those programs was that they were ideal for people using chemicals that were not a part of my world) I set off to get as lean as I could for competition. The only nutritional changes I made were the ones I am having you make. I cut down my intake of fats and sweets, upped my protein intake in relation to my carbohydrates, eliminated complex carbs before bedtime and ate 5-6 meals a day. I lost 30 pounds in 12 weeks while still consuming about 2800 calories a day. I would like to say that I won my competition and lived happily ever after but the truth is I lost too much muscle size because I did too much cardio and lowered my weight training intensity. After my fourth place finish, I kept on my nutrition program for another month but while doing less cardio and again training with greater intensity. After the end of that month, my weight was the same but I was actually leaner because I had gained back some of the lost muscle. The diet program I used was never extreme or caused me to become hungry. It was very different than what a lot of other people were doing for contest prep but I knew then as I know now that there must be an avenue for individual discovery and modification in order for something to be maximally effective and this crude program whet my appetite for finding something that I could present to others for them to utilize for themselves.

Carbohydrate Digestion Rate: One more thing I would like to add about carbohydrates before we move on. Not all complex carbohydrates are created equal. Different carbs have different rates of digestion and absorption into your system. Also, the rate at which they can affect your blood sugar can be different. While this is obviously critical to anyone with diabetic concerns, this can also be of great importance to dieters. Carbohydrates that enter your system rapidly and affects your blood sugar level triggers an insulin release by the pancreas. When these types of carbohydrates are consumed too frequently, the body's sensitivity to insulin can be reduced thus requiring greater insulin output to control blood sugar levels. The excess insulin has the effect of converting the blood sugar or glucose into triglycerides or fats. If you actually get to the point where the pancreas can't produce enough insulin to regulate your blood sugar, then diabetes occurs. Simply put, certain types of carbs, due to faster digestion and assimilation, can be converted to fat a lot faster than other types of carbs. This is exactly what you don't want to happen when you are trying to get leaner.

The Glycemic Index is a scale that was developed that categorizes carbohydrate containing foods by the degree to which they raise your blood sugar levels. Since this **glycotic effect** is also influenced by things like fiber content, water content, protein content and fat content, it is a little more complicated than just complex carbs vs. simple carbs. The bottom line is that your body will react differently to different foods. 40 grams of white potato or white bread will affect you differently than 40 grams of sweet potato or rye bread. That is why, along with the food nutrient list that I provide for you, I also have a list that breaks down a number of well-known carbohydrate foods by their digestion rate. This will give you the ability to fine tune your diet even more and it is a technique I use for my advanced clients and fitness competitors who need to achieve the maximum level of leanness possible. For now, that is not something you need to implement. But I have made it available to you and I will teach you how to utilize it in the final section.

A quick note: One thing I want to point out. Understanding the way our body reacts to certain foods is a very important part of becoming successful in your weight loss program. It may sound logical on paper that "a calorie equals a calorie" and "calories in versus calories out" may seem like a good message for nutritionist to deliver but the body doesn't react that way. Our body is a living organism made up of complex, interrelated systems. You can put two things in a test tube and have those things react upon each other and predict the outcome. You cannot put those same two things in your body and not have them effected by and effect other things. 3000 calories of ice cream, cake, cookies, potato chips and beer will have a dramatically different effect on your body and the way it responds than would 3000 calories of egg whites, chicken breast, brown rice, raw almonds, and spinach. It's not just about reducing calories. It's about giving ourselves the right kinds of calories at the right times. The effect of carbohydrates on our system is a big part of why a lot of people have issues with weight management. That's why we need the right types of foods at the right times. That is also one reason why we should have protein with every meal so that the body (blood sugar level) is less affected by the carbohydrates. And that's one reason why we eat frequent small meals throughout the day so that we are less likely to overload our system at one time with so many calories that our body has no option but to store some of them.

Think of your weight-loss journey just as you would of taking a long trip across country. There is information that you will need in order to accurately arrive at your destination. However, while all the information is important, some of it is relevant only at certain stages of the trip and would just serve to confuse you or lessen your focus on the most meaningful info at other times. For example if you are driving from California to New York to visit Yankee Stadium, you really don't need to start worrying about what freeway exit to take and what side streets to use to get you into the Yankee Stadium parking lot while you are still sitting in your driveway. All you really need to do at that point is start heading in an easterly direction. As you continue, you will fine tune your heading by going northeast and as you get closer to your destination, you will get more and more specific in terms of following the best path. Your weight-loss program should be similar. First you make the basic general changes and then you fine tune with specifics that really allow you to tailor the program to your needs. That is why you don't initially need to worry about carb digestion rates or exact numbers of calories or specific body-fat percentages. These are just tools for fine-tuning the process. But what you will find is that as you progress and learn how your body responds, you will know what it needs and how things will affect you. Once you get to the point where you can actually see the outline of Yankee Stadium, you will know how to get there.

CHAPTER 3

The Secrets of Success

Now that you've learned the basics of structuring your diet some of you may be asking, "Is there an easier way and are there any magical secrets that will make things happen almost overnight?" I will tell you something that many people never learn. **There is no secret, easy way.** Many people, even when they know what they need to do and what will work, instead of utilizing that information to their benefit insist on trying to find a magical shortcut that will circumvent developing good habits. While it is fine to be innovative, there are some basic realities about how the human body works in general and how your body works specifically. The best approach is to utilize the things that are true and will work to create maximum effectiveness. While there are a number of things that can contribute to your success, no one thing by itself can determine your success. That being said, I will tell you that there are some pearls of wisdom and interesting discoveries I've come across over the past 30 years.

1) The Metabolism is the Biggest Key to Continued Success:
We already talked about how some people seem to have it a lot easier than others in terms of how their body utilizes calories. The fact that you are reading this leads me to conclude that you are not one of those people. Welcome to the club! There is good news however regarding those of us with less than ideal metabolic rates. Your metabolic efficiency can be improved and sped up to make it easier for you to get lean and stay lean. The body is always in a constant state of either breaking down or building up. We are either consuming calories, burning calories or storing calories. A lot of this takes place simultaneously. For example, even while you are eating you are burning calories due to various reasons including the digestion process. The importance of this information is for you to

understand that just as "it takes money to make money" it also "takes calories to burn calories".

There is a popular analogy in the fitness industry that is used to illustrate how the metabolism works. If you picture your metabolism as a fire and the food as wood or fuel, you know that by constantly adding small amounts of fuel you will cause that fire to burn hotter and hotter until it reaches its maximum level. If however, you didn't regularly feed the fire, it would die down because it had no fuel to burn. To compound this, if you then threw a large log or "meal" into the already diminished fire, it would not have the capacity to burn it and would be smothered. The body is actually a little worse than this because when the "fire" of your metabolism diminishes it not only has a lessened ability to "burn" food, it also goes into a survival mode, "Oh my god, we must be starving" and proceeds to try its best to store as much of the fuel you give it as possible. Not exactly what we want. That is why eating smaller meals throughout the day is so important.

One of the most useful tools in your weight-loss arsenal is the fact that protein is very thermogenic. Thermogenic substances cause the body to produce heat for energy. All calorie containing substances have thermogenic properties to some degree since calories themselves are merely a way of measuring the heat producing qualities of foods. But protein is particularly thermogenic because unlike fats and carbohydrates it is quite difficult to store as fuel and is not an efficient source of fuel. The work it takes for the body to digest, absorb, and assimilate protein causes the body to expend quite a bit of energy when compared to fats and carbohydrates which give the body easily available energy sources. Now you can see why the first few things we wanted to do with your diet was to cut down the fats and sugars, cut back on excess carbohydrates, up your overall percentage of protein, and increase your eating frequency. Well kept secrets, no. Effective weight-loss nutrition that I have seen work time and time again, year end and year out, yes.

Another metabolic factor is **Body Composition. It's a simple fact that the more lean mass you have the faster your metabolism will be.** Muscle is active tissue that burns calories even in a resting state. That is why you don't want to just lose weight, you want to lose body fat while maintaining or even increasing your lean muscle mass if possible. One of the main reasons that rapid, radical weight-loss programs don't work is that too much muscle tissue is lost as well. Remember, the body prioritizes fat stores for survival purposes and would much rather sacrifice muscle tissue under extreme conditions. It sees muscle as a waste of energy (like not turning off the lights when you leave the room) and when it is in survival mode that is not acceptable. Therefore you can only lose body fat so fast, no matter what some quick fix weight-loss guru might tell you. This amount varies by individual but usually you're looking at only 2-3 pounds of fat loss a week. Don't let this discourage you as this will be a noticeable accomplishment over a period of time. Generally speaking, the slower the weight loss, the more permanent the results. **Better to lose only a couple of pounds a week and keep it off forever than to lose more rapidly only to gain it all back and then be stuck with an even slower metabolism than you had initially because you now have less muscle mass as well.**

I once coached a girl who was getting ready for a fitness competition. Once a week I would check her condition and progress both visually and with calipers. One week she walks in with a big smile on her face, happy that she had lost four pounds since the last time I saw her. She had completely changed the program I had given her, eliminating her weight training and upping her cardio to excessive levels. I knew immediately that she didn't look right and you should have seen the smile disappear from her face once I tested her body fat levels. Despite her four-pound loss, her body fat percentage had actually increased proving she had lost precious lean mass and almost no fat. It was a lot easier to get her to listen to my advice after that. Protecting your lean mass by losing at a controlled and consistent rate will help improve your body composition. Additionally, adequate intake of protein (which we have already covered) plus proper exercise (which we'll soon cover) are also key factors.

2) There is no such thing as Linear Progress: The human body is a dynamic creation that is constantly changing and adapting. It is always trying to reach a point of balance just like a pendulum swinging back and forth striving to reach the center line. Since it operates on so many different variables, it is almost impossible to duplicate the exact same response from the exact same input. That is why there will be weeks when your diet seems to work perfectly and weeks when, having been just as dedicated, you won't experience the same results. One week you may lose two pounds, the next three and the next you may lose nothing or even gain back a pound. This is totally normal in terms of how the body changes and progresses. Don't be discouraged as this is just part of the body's normal adaptation process.

Every time your body changes, you are now dealing with a new set of variables. The "you" that is 15 pounds lighter is different from the previous "you" and therefore will respond differently and have different needs and capabilities. That is why this program is adaptive and allows for periodic adjustments to be made by you. That is also why it is not the worst thing in the world for you to take a break from your normal nutritional regimen and eat some "fun food" on occasion. This actually sends a message to your body that it will not be constantly underfed and that it still needs to maintain its ability to process the maximum amount of calories. This occasional "eating up" as some of my buddies call it can be a very effective tool in helping to maintain an active metabolism, not to mention helping to keep you sane and not overwhelmed by your cravings. Just understand that occasional means just that and you must really monitor the effect of this to make sure that you are not slowing your progress. If you find that your progress is dropping below normal rate, then re-evaluate your diet and make the necessary changes. Refer to the section on breaking out of a sticking point for more specific advice.

3) Set a Goal and Create a Target Date: One of the best things you can do in order to help insure success is to set a goal for yourself to achieve and create a target date for reaching that goal. This is one of the main things successful people do, even if they don't realize it. It is a way of bringing to focus all of your information and effort in order to maximize the effect. Having a specific goal will give a greater sense of purpose to what you are doing. Setting a specific date will serve as an ever present reminder because it will grow closer everyday creating a sense of urgency and keeping you in focus. This is the technique that athletes use to get ready for big competitions. It's the same thing you did as a student when preparing for an important mid-term or final exam. **It's one of the most powerful and effective tools you can utilize to keep yourself on track.**

Try to pick a date or event that already has some significance or meaning to you such as a wedding or class reunion. Failing that, birthdays or holidays also work well. The date should be 12-16 weeks away. If a significant event doesn't exist in this time frame, simply pick a date that would mark the three-month anniversary of you starting on your weight-loss program. The impending arrival of that date serves as a constant reminder and motivator to keep you on track, helping to create a drive that grows to be unstoppable.

The goal you set can actually be quite general. Since people progress at different rates, it is hard to pick a target number in terms of pounds lost that will be accurate enough and it really isn't necessary. Plus, since you might be gaining some muscle, simply stating that you will lose "X" number of pounds might not even be relevant. A good goal would be "I want to get as fit as I can", or "I want to significantly increase my level of leanness". These are appropriate long-term goals that are positive in orientation because you are focusing on improving yourself and adopting the lifestyle and behavior necessary to make those improvements a reality.

During this time frame the possibility of failure doesn't exist, only the opportunity for success. Everyday you get closer to your chance to show the world and yourself what you have accomplished and what you will continue to achieve. **NO ONE OR NO THING CAN STOP YOU!**

4) Have the Proper Mind Set For Weight Loss: For many of you this may be the most important information of this entire program. It is information that I learned from constantly being around people who were in the process of getting leaner week-to-week in pursuit of a goal. **The mindset that it takes for you to successfully**

lose 5-7 pounds is the same mindset that it takes for you to successfully lose any amount of weight that you desire. Think about it, before you can lose 30-40 pounds or whatever, you must first lose that initial 5-7 pounds. In fact, there really isn't a sustainable mindset that will allow you to lose 30-40 pounds. It is too difficult to focus that specifically on such a general goal. I've found that people achieve a lot faster success just by focusing on losing 5-7 pounds and then once that is achieved refocusing on trying to lose the next 5-7 pounds. If you tell yourself that you are going to lose 5-7 pounds by eating better and becoming more active, it is very easy to visualize and believe that you will be successful. If you tell yourself that you will lose 35 pounds or 20 pounds or 65 pounds, chances are you will overwhelm yourself and never even start because there is too much of a part of you that doubts your ability to make it. It just seems too far away. One of the biggest obstacles to overcome is creating a long-term goal that is too intimidating. That is why I advised you to have long-term goals that have more to do with improved overall fitness and health. **It is your short-term goals that will sharpen your drive and create a mindset that leads to success.** And that mindset is to focus on losing the next 5-7 pounds.

Think of it this way. If there were a pile of 100 bricks in your backyard and I asked you to move them into your front yard, there would be no way you could grab them all at once and be able to lift them, let alone carry them around to the front. But you could easily grab one and carry it and then return for another. Sure it would take a while to do this but, without a doubt, if you stuck to it you would eventually finish. People who have had problems with successful weight-loss can best insure success simply by focusing on the short-term goal of losing 5-7 pounds and then repeating that process until they reach their ideal physique. You know you can lose 5 pounds. If you can lose 5 pounds, then you can lose 35 or 45 or 145 pounds if you need to. It's just a matter of focus, knowledge, and time. The only thing I can't give you is the time because you already have it. Remember, time is your friend because it gives you opportunities. It will keep going by whether you choose to utilize it or not. 12 weeks from now will be 12 weeks from now. If you use this time period to implement your program, you will experience 12 weeks worth of progress. And that, for many of you, will be amazing.

5) Always get back on the Horse: Life never has and never will be perfect so there is no reason to expect yourself to be or your diet program to be. If and when things don't go the way you would have liked and you "fall off the horse" don't beat yourself up, just understand that these things happen and get back on the program. Do your best to avoid situations that might be problematic for you. For example, when you're hungry don't go to places where they will have a lot of things that you don't want to eat. It is always OK to bring food with you and one of the big reasons to maintain eating frequency is to help avoid moments of temptation. This is different from when you are allowing yourself to have a special "fun food" meal. I'm talking about a spontaneous situation where you throw all the rules out the window unexpectedly. Unfortunately this happens sometimes. Try to understand the particular set of circumstances that led to this so that they can be avoided next time. Then, simply move forward and refocus on the things you need to do and continue on your way to success. I once had my birthday fall in the middle of my diet for a competition. My girlfriend at the time made me my favorite cake and I "planned" to have just one piece. I thought that I had such willpower and focus that I wouldn't have any problem avoiding it. Needless to say, with that cake there constantly calling my name, my "just one piece" plan went right out the window and evolved into the "as much as you can possibly eat" plan. I wound up having to throw the remainder of the cake out because I would have eventually eaten the whole thing. There was nothing left for me to do but **"get back on the horse"** and refocus on my diet for the rest of the way. Experience taught me that next time I would be better off simply going out for a birthday dessert and then be done with it. We will all make mistakes but life will still go on. Learn from your mistakes so that you don't repeat them and then keep on going and you'll be just fine.

6) Avoid Traps and be Self-Determining: One of the things my little birthday cake incident taught me was the importance of avoiding situations that would leave me vulnerable if at all possible. I call this **"avoiding traps"**. Everyone is different but you must learn which situations are difficult ones for you so that you can be better prepared for them. **Generally when you are on a specific diet, it is not in your best interest to have things around you that may cause temptation**. If you have a weakness for sweets or chips or whatever, you are not doing yourself any favors by having those things stored in your pantry. And when you do decide to break the norm and have something, only purchase what you have pre-allowed for yourself. For example, if I want to have Sun Chips, I will only get the small, individual sized bag. Buying the big "Costco" size bag may be more economical but it will not help you stay on track. I know from my own experience that I would be in that bag on occasion just because it was there. One person I coached had a craving for Oreo's cookies so she decided to indulge. The problem was instead of purchasing the small six-cookie individual pack to satisfy the craving, she bought the large, family size. She was quite upset with herself when in a matter of 2 day's she had wiped out the entire bag. All I could do was give her a hug, make sure she had learned not to put herself into those types of situations in the future and tell her to get back on the horse. A few months later, she had reached all of her goals.

Along with avoiding traps is utilizing **self-determination**. This is where you decide beforehand what you will and will not do, at least for that day or situation. You will be surprised at how well this works. I have actually gone to pizza parties with friends and having previously decided that I would not have any, didn't even feel tempted. A lot of this is mindset, which is different than willpower. Mindset is pre-determined whereas willpower kicks in after you are already "in trouble" and simply trying to resist. As an example I don't drink alcohol but I have a lot of friends who do. I have often heard many of my friends say things like, **"I don't know if I am going to drink tonight,"** before we would head out. Every single time, without fail, they would wind up drinking whether they wanted to or not. What they should have said was, **"I am not going to drink tonight"**. That takes the ambiguity out of it and takes the possibility of them drinking off the table, even if just for that night. The times when my friends took the self-determined approach they didn't seem to have a problem staying with their convictions.

Obviously, you still don't want to frequently put yourself in difficult situations. But, know that you do have a lot of power and control over your actions as long as you understand that you and only you can determine your fate, and you implement and utilize the incredible mind power and resolve that you posses.

I do completely understand that some people are in situations where they have a family or children in the household with them and can't always control what is or isn't within arms reach as far as undesirable foods and beverages are concerned. I think you'll find that the people around you will be quite understanding and willing to be considerate and at least more discrete (like not eating your favorite dessert right in front of you) if you explain your situation to them. And if they are not, that's OK too. It is probably just their own fears and apprehensions about their situation and it will ultimately only increase your resolve. In fact, they are probably admiring you, even when they seem negative, and wish that they had your conviction. Soon you will be an inspiration to them and they will look up to you and may even enlist your help in an attempt to duplicate your success. And helping someone else reach their goals is a wonderful feeling my friend, I can promise you that!

CHAPTER 4

The Importance of Exercise

I will honestly tell you right now that, yes, it is possible to reach all of your weight-loss goals without ever implementing a regular exercise program. **That being said, you will achieve noticeably faster results along with an overall healthier existence simply by incorporating some form of exercise into your life.** It will also give you a lot more control over your look and your ability to maintain your weight-loss once you have reached your goal. Remember when I told you there were no secrets. Well, if there is one secret to effective dieting, it's exercise!

The Center for Disease Control has recently determined that there is a health and fitness crisis existing in the United States and many other parts of the world. According to the government, a poor diet and physical inactivity caused 400,000 deaths in the year 2000, second behind tobacco as a preventable killer. 2 out of 3 adults and over 9 million children are overweight or obese the CDC determined. There is no reason but choice that we need to be part of that group. It is simply a matter of choosing to go in another direction that is a lot healthier and actually quite simple once you get going.

Regular exercise can help prolong your life, combat heart disease, cancer, strokes, relieve stress, create more energy, activate the metabolism, increase your self-esteem, eliminate obesity and make you the sexiest looking dude/chick on the block! Not a bad tradeoff for something that can also be a lot of fun! Plus, there is a feeling of accomplishment that takes places after you exercise, not to mention psychological benefits which are in part due to increased blood circulation and oxygenation of the brain. Physically, mentally, and emotionally, the practice of regular exercise will have a positive effect on your life.

One of the smartest things you can do is to make it a part of your new fitness lifestyle.

Getting Started for Beginners

Doctor's Approval: If you are completely new to exercise or haven't done any form of exercise in quite some time, you should have yourself thoroughly checked out by a medical doctor before going any further. You want to make sure that you don't have any illnesses or conditions than can actually be made worse by exercise, especially if you are significantly overweight. Chances are you will be fine and your doctor will actually encourage you to begin a moderate exercise program, but if you haven't seen a doctor in a while, if there is any chance that you might have some underlying health problem, you really need to make that be your first step. Never put cosmetic success ahead of health concerns. We are talking about creating nothing but positive direction in your life and health so make sure that anything and everything you do takes this into consideration. Once you have been given a clean bill of health from your doctor, then you can start down the magical road of a fitness lifestyle.

Start off Slowly: One very important thing to remember is that you can only change so fast. Therefore, it is never advisable to try and go from doing nothing to doing everything. Your body will adjust best to gradual changes in your activity level as opposed to something that is too taxing or demanding. Remember, if you weren't doing any exercise before, then it won't take much to start effecting changes. You simply need to choose something that is more demanding than your everyday activities and focus it into a structured time frame or schedule so that you can control or regulate your own consistency. It could be utilizing a stationary bike or treadmill, light calisthenics, stretching, or simply walking in place. The biggest key is to choose something that you can do regularly and consistently and that will have enough difficulty that your fitness level must adapt to the challenge.

Enjoyment: Another very important consideration to your exercise program is that you must do something you actually enjoy. If you simply dread doing it, you won't have any problem finding reasons not to. Make your new exercise program as fun as possible. Even if it involves doing a basic, non-exciting activity like walking in place due to lack of equipment, plan your workout so that you are walking while watching your favorite TV show and the time will go by before you know it. I was always amazed at how much cardio I could do when there was a good football game on. It becomes easy to disassociate from any discomfort or fatigue as your attention is elsewhere. Before you know it, you're done!

Exercise is more than just a form of self-inflicted torture. All it takes is a little creativity to make it fun, and that is especially true for cardio. Don't feel like walking around the block, pick up a basketball and shoot some hoop. Imagine how much walking you will be doing chasing down all those missed shots? ☺ And what can be more fun than dancing a few sets at the local dance club for your workout? Remember, if your diet is tight and you're not drinking alcohol while you're there, all your body knows is that it's "movin and groovin" and burning those calories! My good friend Tanya Merryman, Fitness America National Champion, would get in extra workout time by putting on some favorite music and dancing around her living room. That's the biggest benefit of being at a beginning or intermediate level. It doesn't take much to make it work for you. Cycling around the neighborhood, after-dinner walks, or scaling that trusty old staircase 20 times in a row can all form the basis of a workout.

CHAPTER 5

Exercise Types

If your goal is to put together the most ideal and efficient exercise program possible, then there are some important factors to understand. The three main components of fitness are strength training, cardio vascular training, and flexibility. Some training associations refer to this as **"the Fitness Triad"**. There is a relationship and inter-dependency between these components. While they all contribute greatly to overall fitness, too great of a proficiency at one can limit your potential in the others.

Strength and Resistance Training:
Strength for our purposes refers both to the muscle's ability to contract and also the structural strength of the body. Picking up a glass, getting up from a chair, carrying a child, or lifting a weight overhead all require strength. It is an everyday component of our existence that we often take for granted. Strength also exists as our body's ability to withstand the forces of gravity. This can be quite a concern as we get older and battle diseases like osteoporosis. Strength training in some form is ideal for helping to maintain structural integrity by maximizing bone density. In other words, working out not only makes your muscle stronger but also your bones stronger and less brittle. Ironically, one possible benefit that being overweight have given us, due to the extra weight-bearing demands on our structure, is that we might have a head start on bone density and structural strength in some areas, although genetics and nutrition quality are important factors as well. Suffice it to say that some form of strength training whether it's light calisthenics or weight resistance training should be incorporated into your program in order to develop maximum fitness.

There are many benefits to training for ideal strength. First let me state that what is ideal for you may be different for someone else. Everyone needs a base of strength simply to maximize their life and health. You need to have functional strength, or the strength to do your daily tasks without undue effort, like walking up a flight of stairs for example. This doesn't mean you have to start training to become a bodybuilder or a powerlifter. You only need to develop your strength to the degree that it will benefit you and your lifestyle. Basic fitness is a necessity, you need to be able to walk up a flight of stairs. Ideal fitness is our goal. How about walking up those same stairs with a big bag of groceries, while you're talking to your friend on the cell phone and it's no big deal? That could be you!

Strength or resistance training increases the lean mass or muscular development of the body. Generally speaking, the more muscle you have, the faster your metabolism will be. That's why it is important to maintain or even build muscle mass when you are on a fat loss program. **By having that muscle, you will be burning more calories just sitting around doing nothing than you would if you weighed the same or even less with not as much muscle.**

Another benefit of resistance training is that it tends to burn carbohydrates as an energy source. This is ideal for people who have a problem with excess carbohydrate consumption or who simply don't metabolize carbohydrates very well. I have found that a lot of women have trouble in that their bodies tend to store carbohydrates as body fat quite easily. By implementing a good resistance or weight training program their metabolism changes quite noticeably and they become able to achieve and maintain a desired level of leanness a lot more readily. Even if you are not trying to build big, noticeable muscles, if you want to get as lean as possible, as fast as possible, you can do a lot to help your cause by incorporating resistance training.

One final huge benefit of resistance or weight training is post-workout metabolic elevation. Basically, what this refers to is that every time you go through a period of increased activity like a workout, your metabolic rate increases for a period of time, usually for a couple of hours, afterwards. And while this happens to some degree with all workouts, it tends to be most dramatically related to resistance training. This is due to more actual tissue breakdown, greater depletion of energy stores and the need for immediate metabolic recovery by the body. As great as it is to burn calories during the workout, you can imagine the results when you're still burning extra calories a couple of hours after you're done. This type of effect can make a huge difference in your progress. **Remember, it's not how many calories you burn while working out that matters the most, it's how many calories you burn when you are at rest**. Weight training helps this happen in two ways, by increasing lean mass and by elevating the metabolic rate post workout.

Cardio or Aerobic Training: Most of you are already familiar with cardio vascular or aerobic training. It is basically low to moderate intensity training that is done for set time periods with the goal of burning fat for fuel. This is a little different than cardio conditioning which is higher intensity cardio training geared towards developing athletic endurance. Although your endurance will increase to a noticeable degree even from doing low-intensity cardio work, or for that matter resistance work, the primary goal of the type of cardio I will recommend you implement is for accelerated fat burning purposes.

Again, the first thing to do, after you've gotten your doctors approval of course, is to identify your current fitness level and base your workout program on that level. I don't care if you were a marathon runner back in the day, if you haven't worked out for a significant period of time, you need to start out slowly and safely with a beginner type program. As wonderful as cardio training can be, people have the tendency to overemphasize it and do it excessively. Remember rule # 1 of the Kevin principles of cardio: **Don't go from doing nothing to trying to do everything.** If you have been inactive for quite some time, simply walking may be the best thing for you to do. The good thing about cardio training is that it doesn't require specialized equipment to be effective. Walking around the neighborhood or even marching in place can be just as effective as having a $4000 treadmill for a complete beginner. The first thing to consider are pace and time frame.

Start out with a modest goal of 15 minutes a day, three times a week. Go at a pace that allows you to carry on a normal conversation. As this gets easier, you can increase the pace slightly to keep it challenging. After this, increase the duration to 20 minutes for at least two of those days. Once you get to the point where you are doing 20-30 minutes, four times a week, that will be as much cardio as most of you will need to do to make noticeable improvement. Now, here is where I differ from a lot of trainers/coaches. I believe that the majority of people do way too much cardio when they are trying to get into shape. **Your goal shouldn't be to do as much cardio as you can, but as much as you need to!** Unless you are getting ready for some type of physique competition or an athletic event that requires great endurance, you need to really be conscious of doing more cardio than is necessary for you to progress at an ideal pace. Remember, you have to coax your body to change, not force it to change. Four 30-minute sessions of cardio a week is quite a bit. I have seen some girls do an hour plus of cardio a day 5-6 days a week and still look the same or even worse 6-8 months later. That's a whole lot of work for little or no results. So why does this happen?

One thing about the body is that it is geared towards efficiency and is very adaptive. The more cardio you do, the better you get at it and the less beneficial it will be. These girls were simply so good at what they were doing that it wasn't having the desired effect on them. I first noticed this in a number of my friends who were aerobic instructors. They taught 10-12 classes a week and worked out on their own in addition to this and still were not very lean. Not what we want to happen to you. Of course nutrition also plays a huge role. **You can't compensate for consistently poor dietary habits with any amount of activity**. When I'm doing cardio, it takes me about 25 minutes to burn 300 calories. Do you know how quickly I could eat or drink 300 calories even eating clean, let alone eating junk food? One cup of low-fat yogurt is 260 calories. That's why I always tell people, **"It's a lot easier to avoid calories than to burn them!"** People who think they can get lean with tons of cardio to burn off fat and calories are making life a lot harder than it needs to be.

Another side effect of cardio training is that the body starts to adapt to it physiologically as well. Without getting into a long explanation (and believe me I could) basically, your muscle fiber type alters towards more endurance type fibers in terms of size and metabolic rate. In other words you start to lose muscle mass and I'm sure you recall what effect this will have on your metabolism. Again, we are talking about with excessive cardio. The main thing is to implement an effective and beneficial amount without going overboard. One girl I coached was doing 6 days a week of cardio with each session lasting about 45 minutes when she first contacted me. On three of those days, she was actually doing double sessions. The problem was, she still wasn't getting lean and was just about at her wits end. The very first thing I did was to cut her cardio almost in half. Her system was pretty much in shock from all that cardio and her body wanted to hold on to everything. Then I had her up her weight training intensity a little and eat a slightly higher percentage of protein. You should have seen her progress after that. Sometimes it just takes small adjustments to create large changes. Gradually adjust your program and give your body a chance to change and adapt. That's the benefit of invoking a fitness lifestyle. **By consuming less bad calories, the right proportions of quality calories, becoming more active and increasing your metabolic rate simultaneously, small changes are easily managed and can lead to big improvements in your physique.**

For those of you who are reading this that are more advanced you may have gotten to a point where you are used to doing quite a bit of cardio training and feel reluctant to give it up. For a time I provided nutrition services for a cardio kickboxing studio. Many of the women there would take 2-3 classes a day, 5, 6, and even 7 days a week. A number of those same women barley consumed enough calories to sustain themselves. You would have thought that with all the exercise they did and the minimal amount of calories they consumed they would have been quite lean. While a few of them were the majority of them still were not where they wanted to be. They had effectively pushed their metabolisms into survival mode and their bodies were resisting losing any more. For all the time, energy and money they were spending they were stuck and even malnourished in some cases. To make matters worse many of them had lost a fair amount of muscle do to all of this so even the ones without a "weight problem" so to speak were still not as lean and "tight" as they could have been. I was able to convince a few to try a different approach. They started eating more frequently, eating meals with more protein and more total calories, and they implemented weights to help build and/or maintain muscle mass. As the first few started getting good results, more followed. I started to get my own little following but really it wasn't me, it was just a better way of doing things. Some of them turned into my best clients and went on to compete in fitness and figure competitions and do fitness modeling. Others are still there doing the same thing as before, not giving themselves the opportunity to discover that the earth isn't really flat and there is more out there than they've been led to believe. Don't be afraid to keep learning and adapting. Tons of cardio without proper nutrition and in many cases without resistance training won't get it done.

Stretching and Flexibility: It is very important to have a body that is functional and not just attractive. The ability to have and execute movement is something we often take for granted until an injury or illness reminds us of just how precious it is. I am sure most of us have at times had a stiff back or neck and recall how difficult even the most simple of tasks can quickly become. That is why it is always good to implement some type of regular stretching and flexibility training into your fitness program. I'm not talking about trying to become a contortionist or a member of the Chinese acrobatic team. I am simply talking about a regular attempt to maintain spinal flexibility, as well as joint and muscular flexibility. Personally, I like to do some light stretching as part of my warm-up program and continue doing a little more aggressive stretching while I am actually in between sets during my resistance program (Yes, I know some research shows that this can effect maximum power out put but since I'm not a powerlifter I'd rather sacrifice a little strength if necessary for added safety and longevity). Another great time for stretching is at the end of your workout when everything is nice and warm. This is great for recovery, relaxation, and works as an effective cool down. It is also the best time to work on your flexibility since you are already warm and considerably more elastic if that is a goal. The main point though is to develop and maintain efficient body movement and function for health and fitness benefit. Although I am limited in what I can teach you here there are many avenues available to you to learn more about stretching in order to incorporate it into your program. And if you choose to follow flexibility based holistic training like yoga or Pilates, I think those are excellent avocations in which to involve yourself. Remember, just like any new physical activity, always start off safely and conservatively. Stretch initially only to the point of positive sensation and comfort, never to the point of pain or possible injury. Stretching should actually feel good as it will be energizing and help increase circulation. It is an excellent way to get back in tune with your body and start developing that mind/body link that is so beneficial to achieving ultimate fitness. Having and maintaining proper flexibility will also help with injury prevention if you decide to get involved with sports participation during your fitness program. In these instances you will be incorporating both general, overall body stretching and specific area stretching. For example, I always do basic core stretches before my workouts and then do additional stretching for the body parts I am training, like hamstrings for example, throughout the course of the workout. It will take some exploration and experimentation to develop your ideal stretching program but the main thing is to understand that the inclusion of regular stretching and mobility work is an important ingredient in the recipe for optimal fitness.

CHAPTER 6

Tips for Success

Even if you are not new to the world of fitness and working out, there are still a number of fitness tips that you may not be familiar with that can greatly improve your success. While it is true that everyone is to some degree unique, there are researched and documented findings about how the body responds to exercise that can be implemented to improve your fitness results. **One rule of thumb that I always go by is to never discount anything that you know to be true about your body**. There are simply things that don't apply to you the same as everyone else and if you have had a lot of success with a certain method or philosophy, by all means don't alter it just because some "expert" all of a sudden tells you it is wrong. Always take any new information and add it to what you already know to increase your knowledge level. And if two seemingly conflicting ideas are presented, keep an open mind and understand that there is more than one way to do certain things and that another way might work better for someone else than it has for you. Remember, anyone can give advice. But not only should they be able to tell you what to do, but also why you should do it. And if they really know their stuff, they should be able to tell you why you should do A as opposed to B,C,D,or E. You can be sure that advice at this level is coming from a knowledgeable person who is taking into consideration your best interests and your individual needs. I have often been amused when I would design a program specifically for someone based on every factor in their life and some "trainer" who knew only limited ways to do things and nothing about my client's goals would challenge them on their approach simply because it wasn't what they themselves had learned to do.   A lot of people only learn one way to do things when in fact, there is always the possibility for improvement. That is why I went through certification courses with two companies that were philosophically at opposite ends of the spectrum and I used my over three decades of personal experience and observation to figure out the useful information from the less than useful information in terms of what to pass on to others. With that in mind, here are some fitness and workout tips that I offer for your consideration and meditation:

Make a Commitment to Yourself and Your Program: The best way to insure success is to become as consistent as possible. The only way for you to develop this consistency is to commit yourself completely. Decide in advance what your workout schedule will be and stick to it no matter what. If you decide that you are going to workout on Monday, Wednesday, and Friday at 6:00PM then, come hell or high water, that's what you will do and don't let anything or anyone get in the way of your plans. By committing to a specific time and schedule you will develop discipline. You owe it to yourself to stick to your commitment to make the changes that you want. This is something that you are doing for yourself because you want to and you deserve the benefits that will result. Ultimately fitness will become second nature to you and you will always make time to include it in your life but initially it will always seem as if something else is competing for your fitness time so you must be extra diligent in prioritizing your goals and yourself. Treat it as a responsibility the same as you would treat going to work or going to class. You commit to those activities because you value the results, rewards, or knowledge. **The results of committing to your fitness program will have a value that far exceeds anything you have ever experienced and you owe it to yourself to make it happen.**

Enjoy and Improve: In order for you to stay with your workout program long enough for it to be successful, there are two things that you must get from your training. You have to enjoy your workout experience and you have to be making progress and seeing improvement. If you only have one of these factors it will be difficult for you to make it work. If you are enjoying your training but not making progress, sooner or later you won't be able to justify to yourself the amount of time you spend doing the activity. If you are making improvement but not having any fun, you risk becoming bored and it will be too easy for you to find something else to do instead. Try to pick activities that are challenging but still fun. Working out doesn't have to be something that you dread doing. Sure, there will be moments of effort, sacrifice, and discomfort, but not to the extent that it deters your motivation. In fact, you will probably find yourself inspired by the fact that you were able to physically accomplish something that was not possible for you just a short time ago. Keep a positive attitude about your training and incorporate activities that are fun and enjoyable whenever you can and you will be amazed by the momentum you begin to build.

Do your cardio right when you get up in the morning or immediately after your weight training: The reason for this is that you will burn a higher percentage of stored body fat when your blood sugar is low and your own glycogen stores are depleted. If you do your cardio training before your weight work, your body will have a greater amount of glycogen (stored carbohydrates) available for energy and it will take longer before it accesses your fat stores. By doing your weight work first, you reduce your muscle and liver glycogen and your blood glucose levels and your body is forced to dip into your fat stores sooner and to a greater extent when you do your cardio. This condition exists somewhat naturally in the morning due to the amount of time you've been fasting (especially if your last food meal contained no complex carbs) so it is an ideal time to effectively do cardio. You don't have to have a completely empty stomach as many people believe. It is OK to eat some light-protein to keep the old stomach from growling while you put in your morning session.

It is better to do two 30 minute sessions of cardio in one day than to do one 60 minute session: A lot of people like to do really long cardio sessions as we discussed earlier. If you want to do more cardio, it is actually more effective splitting the sessions into two shorter sessions. This will give you two times a day that you give your metabolism a boost and also experience the post workout metabolic increase that I mentioned earlier. Also, by avoiding excessively long cardio sessions, you will avoid burning up that precious muscle tissue which keeps your metabolism active. So if you find yourself getting to the point where you want to add more cardio and you are already at 30-40 minutes a session, consider adding a separate session at another time of day like in the morning or post-workout. Then you can increase the intensity of those 30-40 minute sessions to keep them progressive. That higher intensity will lead to even greater post workout metabolic activation.

Another option for the more advanced is to do shorter, more intense cardio sessions like 20 minutes of interval training. This is where you do a warm-up then follow with periods of higher intensity cardio alternated with low-intensity recovery periods. This is quite effect for losing body fat and maintaining muscle while really boosting the metabolic rate. The point is that simply doing more and more cardio for longer and longer periods of time is not the best approach for most trainees and will not give you your best results.

Not all weight-loss is the same: There is a difference in the amount of effort and time it will take between losing your first five pounds and your last five pounds. What I mean by this is that the greater amount of excess body fat you have, the easier it will be to lose compared to after you've gotten leaner when it will be more difficult to get rid of. This is something you need to understand in terms of why your progress will most likely slow down. When you first start your program, at say 40 pounds overweight, your body has quite an excess of stored adipose tissue (fat) and isn't all too concerned when it starts to lose it. As your body-fat percentage lowers and you have less overall fat to lose, your body will place a higher priority on holding onto your fat stores and make losing fat not quite as easy as it initially was. Add to that the fact that you are probably now in better shape and it takes greater effort to effectively produce changes and you can see why your progress will often slow. The key is to understand that this is quite normal and just calls for some adjustments on your part. Refer to my section on overcoming sticking points for more info. The good thing is that the changes you make at this point in time will have a much more dramatic effect on your overall look and really bring about the finishing touches to your physique. Losing that first 5-10 pounds may not appear as dramatic but losing that last 5-10 pounds can really take you to another level.

One bit of important advice I want to add. Always remember that the body can only change and only lose fat so fast. If not we could simply stop eating for two weeks, do 8-10 hours of cardio a day, drop 30 pounds and be done with it, right? Obviously it doesn't work this way as I mentioned before because your body prioritizes survival first and is always trying to protect you. Therefore, if you try to lose too fast your body will not exceed its natural fat loss limits but will simply start losing muscle due to the energy crisis it will consider itself under. One of the biggest mistakes people make is trying to lose too fast and when they do they are sacrificing their metabolic rate. If you do this you make it very difficult to reach your goals because before you get all the way there, your body will become quite stubborn and will began to fight you. Many times when people are first starting out and weight loss is easiest it is also more difficult to determine if you are losing fat, muscle, or both. Consequently they lose too fast as they are of the mindset that just losing weight (as opposed to getting leaner) is all they need to do. They are making long term progress more difficult and increasing the chance that they will rebound and gain it all back. Having been in the fitness industry for so long I have had the opportunity to really observe people over the long term. I have seen many occasions where people were so excited with the changes they made (having lost 40-50 pounds) only to see them a year or two later quite depressed and seemingly defeated once they had gained it all back (and then some!). Sure some people may be able to get away with rapid changes, at least for a while, but generally speaking slow and steady will ultimately provide a lot better results. It is much more of a marathon than a sprint. Stay patient and do things the right way and the healthy way. Your body will thank you in the long run.

Lift to build not to get smaller: The reason that you should be doing resistance or weight training is to build your muscles. This will add strength and shape to your body as well as tone and hardness. You can use this type of training to balance your physique and develop ideal symmetry and proportions plus elevate your metabolic rate. Often I see people with very light weights doing an exercise in an attempt to reduce the size of the area they are working. Mistakenly they think they are developing "tone" when the truth is that the resistance they are using is so light it is having virtually no effect at all. If you have an area that you feel is too big like your arms or legs for example, chances are it's not the muscles that are too big, it's that the area is not yet lean enough. The purpose of training this area is to develop the muscle that is underneath so that when you get leaner you have a nice, firm physique. In order to do this you need to use sufficient resistance, enough to challenge the muscle and cause form failure in the 8-15 repetition range. If you feel that a particular muscle is indeed too large, simply don't work it because if you have an area that grows that easily, (extremely rare) even light resistance work could keep it from reducing in size. Generally what I see are people training with weights as if their muscles were too big and they are trying to make them smaller when in fact all they really need to do is just get leaner. With the right diet, cardio for accelerated fat burning, and proper resistance training for ideal muscle development, they will soon have a lean, low-fat, toned physique.

If you find that weight training does cause you to grow faster than you would like simply decrease the rest periods between sets. This way you can train with enough intensity to effect the metabolism and keep the muscle density (tone) but since you are only resting 30-45 seconds in between sets you won't be able to use sufficient enough weight (if you keep the rep range at 12-15) to really cause too much of a size increase.

Do as much as you need to not as much as you can: Whether it's resistance training, cardio, or dieting your goal is to do an effective amount to stimulate positive change, not spend all of your waking hours in the gym. Exercise and a fitness lifestyle are very positive things and if everything clicks perfectly for you it will be a fun and fantastic journey. But be careful not to let your enthusiasm get the best of you and cause you to overextend yourself. Your body can only change so rapidly and no amount of training or dieting beyond what is necessary will alter that. People whose programs are excessive are a lot more susceptible to injury or illness and they may eventually experience the phenomenon of diminishing returns for their efforts. It has been my experience observing the "workoutaholics" that they are more likely to burn out on what they are doing and wind up spending extended periods of time away from the fitness lifestyle. Pace yourself in your training and implement a schedule that you can permanently fit into your life as opposed to one that you will be struggling to maintain a few weeks or months down the road.

When you have to choose make the best choice: Many times you will find yourself in situations where your normal plan gets tossed out the window and you are forced to adapt. At times like this, don't allow frustration to cause you to sway from your overall philosophy and beliefs. Simply make the best choice available to you under the given circumstances that will most reflect what it is you wish to accomplish. If this means making a selective choice from a fast food restaurant or having to modify a planned workout because you are completely out of time, just get through it as best you can and realize that an occasional bump in the road won't stop you from arriving at your destination. Use this as a learning experience and incentive to pre-plan for unexpected situations whenever possible. Most fast food places have healthy menu items that will work just fine for you. And having to helter skelter a workout every once in awhile can really keep the body guessing. Here's a side tip, when you find that you don't have time for your full workout and you have to choose between doing weights or cardio, most often you will be best off doing the weights. A weight training workout will burn just as many or more calories as a cardio workout plus have the added effect of elevating your post-workout metabolism to a greater degree and for a longer period of time. Add to this the fact that by limiting your between sets rest period (remember you are short on time) you will be receiving a cardio vascular benefit anyway and you can see why this might be your best choice. I recall reading an article by former Ms. Met-Rx Tara Phillips (Caballeros) and how she had always prioritized her cardio and aerobic training. Once she made the switch to regular resistance training she was finally able to get the results she had been looking for and if she ever found herself with only a half an hour to workout, she would choose to do her weight training over her cardio because she felt that this would help her maintain the lean mass that contributed so much to her very successful look. For many reasons I agree with Tara and it's definitely something for you to consider if you ever find yourself in that situation as opposed to just automatically doing nothing but cardio. This would tend to be even truer if you find you must make this choice for an extended period of time as doing only cardio could cause you to lose enough lean mass to negatively effect both your body composition and your metabolic rate.

For the record: Some of you may be wondering if it is ever OK to only do cardio for your workout and not include any resistance training? Of course it is, especially if you are a beginner and are just trying to up your activity level in conjunction with your new dietary habits in order to lose weight. I certainly don't want to give you the impression that I am "anti-cardio". You can accomplish many things through dietary manipulations alone and adding any good workout program just makes things that much better. If you have an aversion to resistance training or feel that it just isn't something that would be right for you, don't feel pressured into trying it or start believing that you won't be successful without it. I am merely telling you what I feel is the best possible way for both short-term and long-term success to give you the most noticeable and lasting results. I'm sure a lot of people reading this have experienced a degree of success when following other programs but for some reason the results didn't continue and you either stopped short of your goal or even reverted back to your previous situation. The information I am giving you is the best information to get you all the way to your greatest imagined goals and keep you there forever. That is why I am offering you information that may be a little more geared towards changing your previous behavior and offering you new information to consider and implement. Remember, one of the first things I said is that you have to be willing make a change if you want things to be different. So, while what I tell you may not be the only way, I am committed to helping you find what I believe to be the best way and the best way is to adopt fitness as a lifestyle approach that incorporates proper nutrition and diet combined with the major components of exercise; cardio training, resistance training, stretching, and proper rest and recovery.

If it sounds too good to be true: Did you really think that eating bacon/cheese burgers was the best way for most people to get as lean and fit as possible just because they didn't eat the carbohydrate containing bread? How about attaching electrodes to your muscles and using a current to stimulate new growth? Or what about that workout course or machine that you only have to do 5-7 minutes a day for 30 days to have washboard abs, rock hard glutes and star in the next James Bond movie? Hey, I completely understand marketing. And I am not saying there isn't merit to a lot of the things that you see advertised in the media today. But some of those companies are just down right lying to you. Even worse, some of them are being completely irresponsible by promoting dietary philosophies that could be very unhealthy and harmful to you. No I am not a doctor, but any doctor who signs off to endorse a product or diet program that is high in saturated fat, low in fiber and may lead to heart disease and obesity problems in order to profit, at the potential expense of your health, should not be allowed to call himself/herself a doctor either! It is not just about how you look but about how healthy you are!

Now there are some excellent products and pieces of equipment on the market. Most companies use fitness models (a number of which who are personal friends of mine) to help get your attention and effectively advertise their products. I am completely fine with this as long as you understand that the models endorsing these products looked like that long before most of these products even existed. That's why they were selected to endorse these products in the first place. And they achieved their look by following a fitness lifestyle very similar to the one I am recommending for you. If a particular product you see advertised is advocating, teaching, or making it possible for you to practice a fitness lifestyle, then it may very well be an excellent product for you to consider. If the product you see advertised is trying to lead you away from the path of health and fitness by promoting some easier alternative, remember what I said about there being **"no secret and easy way"**. Always use your best judgment and try not to get caught up in the hype. The more you continue to learn about health and fitness and practice a fitness lifestyle, the easier it will be for you to recognize what types of things will benefit your physical well being and what types of things will not.

Get help if you need it: Some people thrive on doing things alone or figuring things out for themselves. Other people tend to do better with assistance and take help whenever they can get it. Either way is fine as long as you are doing what is best for you. But it is important to understand that if you are having trouble figuring out something on your own, it is perfectly OK to get help if you need it. Help can come in a number of different forms. You are getting help with your fitness lifestyle right now simply by reading this. If you find you need more help in certain areas, it is available as well. When I first started working out, I learned to do a lot of the weight training exercises simply by reading books and magazines that contained exercise descriptions with pictures. That was all that really existed back then. Now, you also have CD-ROM, video, DVD's, personal trainers, online training and nutrition programs, websites, and I'm sure a few knowledgeable friends and co-workers to help guide you along. Use whatever source you feel is necessary and best for you. Actually, I would suggest utilizing more than one reference/educational source when it comes to exercise description and technique to avoid being limited to any one particular point of view. Personal trainers can be great if you can afford one, at least for a few workouts until you learn what you need to know. The key is to find a trainer who will teach you what you need and focus on your goals as opposed to trying to sell you on more sessions and/or withhold information to keep you dependant on them. Not that there is anything wrong with having someone train you regularly, I think that is a great way to progress if that's what you want to do. Trainers can also be great for added motivation and helping you stay committed and on track. But they should understand that their role is to assist you in achieving your goals, not to take over any aspect of your life. If all you want is for someone to teach you how to correctly do the basic exercises, design a program for you, and then let you do your thing, then you want them to understand that you're not interested in their sales pitch and if you need more info you'll contact them again. That being said there is really no substitute for having a knowledgeable and experienced person working with you to help you achieve your goals. You can learn exercise techniques, have specific questions answered, receive encouragement and motivation, and always have that someone in your corner who cares about you and your progress if you have a good trainer.

I considered writing up some basic workout routines for this book and including them for you but with so many different levels of people who might be reading this from very beginners to quite experienced veterans it would be impossible to accurately and responsibly cover everything in a way that would fit everyone's needs both safely and effectively. And while I could live with knowing that maybe some readers might consider what I wrote as not being specific enough to really benefit them, I would have ongoing concerns about someone trying something that was maybe a little beyond their current capabilities and becoming either frustrated or, even worse, getting injured because they were following a generalized program I wrote up that was never intended for them. When I design a program for someone, the first thing I have them do is fill out an extensive questionnaire that gives me a lot of information about their level of experience, goals, time availability, workout and injury history, potential risk factors, motivation, etc. There is no way to generalize a program or group of programs in this format with any degree of accuracy or responsibility. But the thing about learning from others, me or anyone else, is that you learn what they choose to teach you and what they deem to be important. This is an opportunity for you to learn some things that you feel are important and that excite and motivate you. Go to the bookstore, browse the internet, buy a few magazines, tour a health club or two, talk to your friends, and just see what's out there. Most of what I learned I had to specifically pursue but it was out there and I did find it. From college courses and every book and magazine I could find, to certification courses and exchanging viewpoints with my fellow gym rats and fitness enthusiast, if it was out there and could help me, I found it. Hopefully, I am saving you a lot of time by condensing the best of what I discovered through time, effort, trial and error, and I am setting you up to have maximum success and enjoyment in the shortest possible time with a minimum amount of frustration. So go out there and explore for both knowledge and enjoyment, it will only add to your experience.

Home Training Versus Gym Training: You may be wondering if it would be better for you to workout at home or to join a gym or health club in order to achieve the best results. The truth of the matter is that either can be effective and it really comes down to what you would be most comfortable with. Obviously, a well equipped gym will have advantages in terms of variety and diversity of quality equipment, but as long as you have what you need, you can accomplish just as much training at home. Home training can be quite convenient and really only requires a minimal amount of equipment. Truth be told, you can do an effective workout without any commercial equipment if you have the right knowledge level and attitude. In terms of effective variety and motivation I would at least recommend some type of cardio equipment and some adjustable resistance equipment, but depending upon your level and your goals, it really is all about what you want to do and how you want to do it. If you do decide to purchase workout equipment however, I would recommend purchasing equipment of the highest quality that you can effectively budget. Very often beginning workout enthusiast buy the cheapest equipment available with the philosophy that they want to first see if they will utilize it before investing a greater amount. The problem is that cheap equipment is often cheaply made and frequently doesn't feel quite right when you are using it which will greatly effect your motivation and your results. Not to mention the fact that it is often constructed from materials that don't last so even if you do use it regularly, you will be replacing it long before you thought you would. Higher quality equipment looks better, feels better, and is a lot more fun to use which, as I mentioned earlier, is an important factor in your ultimate success. Plus, if you purchase quality equipment and you ever deicide that you no longer have a use for it, it will not be that difficult to find an interested buyer for it as opposed to low-quality equipment which no one will want. Even if you start off working out at home and then join a great gym, you will still find plenty of days when it is just a nice option to be able to jump on your home treadmill or knock off a 20-minute weight workout without leaving the house.

Of course one benefit of training at a gym or health club is the potential motivation you can receive by being in an environment where others are working on goals of self-improvement just like you. And don't forget that the social interaction with other gym members can make for a more enjoyable fitness lifestyle. While it was never my original intention, I must admit that I have made some wonderful friends at the gym including my best friend and my business partner and I can't imagine how different my life would be without these associations. There is a certain degree of apprehension and insecurity when entering an unfamiliar arena, especially for beginners. I recall when I was managing Gold's Gym how people would tell me they were too intimated to come there because they thought it would be too hardcore and they were not fit enough. Any gym or health club that takes the approach that a potential member is not fit enough to belong will very soon be out of business. The fact of the matter is new members are extremely valuable and desired and the club ownership and staff should be willing to do everything possible to make you feel at home and to help you achieve success so that you become a long-term member and basically a walking advertisement for the quality of their facility. It's not at all about whether or not they want you, but whether or not you want them. Just remember to shop around and see if you feel comfortable. Make sure that if you do join and don't like it for any reason, you can always quit and go somewhere else. If they only offer contracts, then chances are once they have your enrollment fee and are regularly getting your money they don't care anymore about you because they will be getting paid whether you show up or not. As long as you avoid that type of situation, any good club will want to be very in-tune with maximizing your fitness experience and maintaining your business.

Supplements: Good or Bad? There is a lot of confusion, debate, and misunderstanding involving the nutritional supplement industry. Supplements have been praised and credited with producing miraculous results and also condemned and accused of being poisonous snake oils. Which is true? Neither one of course. A supplement can be either effective or ineffective depending upon what it is, how it is used, and what results are expected from it. The problem is that they can be just as easily misused if there is a lack of knowledge by the user or that user is mislead by someone with regards to that supplement. First of all, supplements should be just that, something taken to supplement your normal dietary habits. They are not meant to take the place of good nutritional practices. They are intended to be used in addition to quality foods and beverages, not instead of them. Basically, there are two types of supplements; food supplements and performance enhancing supplements. Food supplements are concentrated parts of foods or food substances that are used to add extra amounts of that particular food item to the diet to either combat a deficiency or to fulfill a need. Generally they are taken to support the natural processes of the body. Examples of these are; protein and meal replacement powders, vitamins and minerals, fluid and electrolyte replacement drinks, and digestive enzymes. Performance enhancing supplements are food or herbal concentrates, extracts, or tinctures that are used in an attempt to promote a response from the body or endocrine system that is optimal or at least greater than its normal activity. This would include things like creatine monohydrate, beta alanine, L-glutamine, caffeine and the recently banned herbal stimulant ephedra. It would be an oversimplification to say that food supplements are safe and effective and performance enhancing supplements are dangerous and non-effective.

Proper supplementation can help add nutritional insurance in support of an ideal or optimal eating plan. Many experts believe that humans can obtain all the nutrients they need through the foods they consume and therefore have no need to supplement or consume things like vitamins and minerals. The problem is that too often, due to restrictive or unbalanced eating, poor food quality, or increased biological need due to stress, pollution, or other environmental concerns, it is possible to become deficient in one or more nutrients. Also, there is a debate over what amount of certain nutrients the human body really needs. Standards like the RDA's (recommended daily allowance) were developed decades ago (in the 1930's) and the amounts recommended were the minimum amounts of certain nutrients known to be necessary to keep healthy humans free of certain specific diseases (like vitamin C to prevent scurvy and vitamin D to prevent rickets). But there is a big difference between the minimum amount of something you need just to keep from becoming ill and the optimal amount your body should have in order to develop peak health and vitality. Along with consuming a wide variety of fresh and unprocessed foods including whole grains, fruits, vegetables, seeds, nuts, dairy, leans meats, fish, eggs, and poultry, many people still find it beneficial to include additional supplements for nutritional insurance. A good vitamin and mineral supplement that includes anti-oxidants and digestive enzymes is something that at least should be considered by most active people.

Problems arise with supplementation when misuse or overuse occurs due to a lack of knowledge or understanding as to what a product can and cannot do. Many people tend to extrapolate the potential effect of a supplement and quickly get carried away with its use, ignoring the instructions or recommendations on the bottle. The product ephedra was a great example of this type of situation because as soon as people heard that it might be an effective weight-loss aid, it quickly became overused by a great many people who never stopped to consider what it really was and potential problems it might cause even though these were listed right on the label. There are times when people need to be protected from themselves and since quite a number of people were actually abusing a product that was not intended to be used in excess, it was in my opinion a good idea for it to be removed from the market. As a rule of thumb, you should never use any supplement or drug unless you know everything you possibly can about it, what it will and will not do, what potential side effects it might have, and exactly how it is to be used. And even if you do know this information any new product should be used as directed and with caution and responsibility. Ephedra was a product that was not used or marketed responsibly resulting in problems for some individuals and the entire supplement industry.

There has never been and probably will never be a supplement or drug that can do more for an individual's ability to develop and maintain ideal weight, health, and fitness than proper nutrition, exercise, and time. The use of weight-loss pills, potions, and formulas should be secondary to the implementation of a proper diet and fitness lifestyle. The majority of people will find that lifestyle changes will make the perceived need for some form of outside dietary assistance non-existent. The use of supplements to support an ideal nutritional program can be very beneficial but people should always be wary of products that promise to give results without addressing the need to make more relevant and beneficial changes.

On a personal note I have used quite a few nutritional supplements over my fitness career. I have been taking multiple vitamins and minerals for over 30 years. I have used a number of protein powders and meal replacement drinks and have tried performance enhancing products like creatine monohydrate and various pre and post workout formulas from some of the top supplement companies in the industry. I would have to say that I have had good experiences with the things I have used and have received favorable nutritional support for my training and nutrition endeavors. I honestly believe that if you are seriously hard in training then the right additional nutrients can be a beneficial aid to energy, recovery, and overall progress. But also understand that I have been very dedicated and consistent in my training and nutrition practices. I have also never smoked, drank alcohol, or used either recreational or performance enhancing drugs. First and foremost you must get the basic diet and eating patterns correct before you can determine if there will be a need for supplementation. And if you are not physically active you may not ever get to a point where your body needs additional nutritional support. First optimize the diet and exercise program, only then will you be able to truly benefit from supplementation. And if you do decide to give them a try stick with name brand reputable companies whenever possible. There's a reason these companies have been in existence for a while. They have a lot at stake to put out quality products that people can use with confidence and rely on. If a particular supplement is of value, you can be sure that the majority of the big name companies will carry it (or some version of it if it's something like a pre-workout formula or fat burner). With some of the newer companies I have found that their focus is more on making a buck and not on the integrity of the industry or the well being of their customers. They will market borderline items or associate drug-like results to common or unproven items simply to win over new customers. Some of these companies don't care about doing things the right way as they don't plan on being around that long. They simply want to make the money and run. Put your trust in companies that have either been around awhile and/or are doing things in such a way that it's easy to see they plan to. Never put anything in your body unless you can have a pretty good understanding and confidence about what it is, what it does, and how to use it.

Medical Procedures, Drugs, and Medications for Weight Loss:
There are many options and choices when it comes to weight-loss including the use of drugs, medications, and surgical procedures. The lure of a possible quick and easy solution may seem difficult to resist but the truth of the matter is that there is usually nothing quick or easy about any medical procedure. Any decisions involving using medication or surgery as an answer to being overweight should be well informed and well thought out by both you and your doctor. All the potential risks and side effects should be thoroughly explained, discussed, and considered before any decisions are made. If your health or life is at risk, you really need to listen to everything your doctor tells you and together decide what would be the best thing for you to do in order to get better. If you are in a situation where remaining overweight puts you at a risk that is greater than medical intervention and that risk is imminent, then your doctor may determine that the best thing for you is a surgical procedure or medication. If there is no immediate health risk and the medical options are just seemingly more convenient, you really need to stop and consider if this is truly the best choice for you. There are a lot of factors that can contribute to being overweight including; biological, behavioral, genetic, and psychological. It is to your benefit to educate yourself fully as to any options you might be considering outside of adopting a fitness lifestyle and to enlist competent and objective advice whenever possible by someone who has nothing but your best interest at heart.

One of the most dramatic of all medical procedures for weight-loss is gastric bypass or stomach stapling. This is the surgical procedure that reduces the size of the stomach to such a degree that the patient becomes physically unable to eat more than a minute amount of food at a given time. This is a major, life altering procedure in more ways than one and, like any proposed change to your body, needs to have all of its potential implications weighed not only for weight-loss purposes but for lifestyle purposes as well.

I recall one day about six-months after I had left my position as manager of Gold's Gym. I was managing a high-end exercise equipment store in Northern Ca. that is owned by a friend of mine called All American Fitness. A gentleman came into the store and walked up to me with a big smile on his face. I immediately recognized him as someone I knew pretty well but for some reason, the details, including his name, were escaping me. We started small talking about how long it had been since we'd seen each other and he introduced me to his daughter. As I continued to listen to his very familiar voice, it finally dawned on me who he was and that it was shock that was clouding my memory. Oh my God, it was my friend Mark Powell who I hadn't seen in about two years. As I explained to Mark that I recognized him but it took a minute to register, his grin grew even broader for he was quite used to this reaction. The last time I had seen Mark, he weighed in the neighborhood of 400 pounds. Now, here he stood looking like a new person at around 220. This was a pretty substantial change for Mark who was a friend I knew from Gold's and stood 5'8 in height. Ever since I met Mark, he was always a big guy. He had actually been a competitive power lifter and wrestler in his youth and when I knew him at Gold's he was still one of the strongest guys in the house. I remember that Mark's weight had gotten to be pretty noticeable but it was never something that we addressed and to me he was just Mark, always happy, always strong, and one of the nicest guys in the place. He told me that after I left (I went to manage another gym for the same ownership) his weight had gotten to be more and more of a problem and his eating had gotten out of control. He said he got up to about 420 pounds and didn't see any way to stop it when the light of reality finally came on and he realized that his life was at risk. There were certain things that happened within his family emotionally that triggered Mark's enlightenment, but the bottom line is that there came a time when he could no longer live in denial about the fact that he was not where he wanted and needed to be and made the decision to do something about it. Because Mark's situation had gotten to a medically critical point and he needed to actually insure that he would not gain any more weight, on the advice of his doctor, he opted to have a gastric bypass procedure. This stopped the out-of-control weight increase that Mark felt he was experiencing but there still was a lot of work to be done. Mark made his way back to the gym and resumed his workouts, this time with another goal. He started doing regular walking along with his weight lifting in order to help lose body fat faster. When walking became easier, he started jogging a little, gradually increasing the length and pace as he got into better and better shape. Mark's physique began to change quite noticeably due to the radical change in calories and the increased activity levels. Mark didn't just lose weight, he made himself into a fitter and more healthy person. The 220 pound Mark that stood smiling before me was still able to bench press over 500 pounds and now had the energy to coach his high school age son in wrestling and help him practice as well as keep up with his beautiful teenage daughter. Being able to spend positive time with his kids, both now and in the future, was no small motivation for Mark to get back to being healthy and fit. And even though he was practically forced to have a very radical procedure due to immediate health concerns, he instantly knew that his ultimate success was still in his hands and that it was necessary to incorporate a fitness lifestyle again to really maximize this new chance that he had been given. Mark's is a wonderful and still ongoing story and I had the pleasure of interviewing him and hearing much of it. I will save that for him to tell you in his own way and in his own time. But what I want you to take away from this is that even if you do choose medication, liposuction, gastric bypass, psychological counseling, or whatever, if you are still physically capable of adopting a fitness lifestyle, I think you will find that it will help you complete the process and ultimately find yourself.

CHAPTER 7

Overcoming Sticking Points

Progress that stops: It is quite normal to be rolling along just fine with your weight-loss program then all of a sudden it just doesn't seem to be working anymore. Worse still is to lose a significant amount and then almost without notice, you are heading in the other direction. How do you keep the progress going and how do you keep from gaining back the weight you worked so hard to get rid of? The first step is not to panic. Remember what I said earlier about linear progression and how it doesn't exist? It is perfectly normal for your bodyweight to fluctuate. Gaining weight doesn't mean that you've gained back unwanted body fat. The first important step is to stay constantly aware of what your body is doing. Don't let yourself slip back into the old habit of living in denial. As much as you might not want to acknowledge that you've just gained 10 pounds, having that knowledge is a whole lot better than burying your head in the sand and not pulling it out until you've gained back 30 or 40 pounds. Maintaining your awareness, whether you are gaining back or simply no longer losing at the desired rate, allows you to maintain your control and make the changes necessary to get you going in the right direction again.

Finding the Problem: The first step is to re-check your eating habits. This means that if you have stopped writing down everything you are consuming then it is time to start keeping track again. This will tell you right away if there are any obvious bad habits that you have the ability to alter to get yourself back on track. It also gives you back the accountability and re-sharpens your focus. If everything seems to be on track nutritionally, look to your activity level. Have there been any recent changes that could be affecting the number of calories you're burning in a day? Did you change to a more sedentary job? Did you take a break from working out or cut back on your program? Are you less active outside due to a change in the weather? Any of these things could account for having slowed your progress. If there are no obvious differences in either your nutrition or activity level, your body may have simply reached a set-point for your current program and it is time to make some adjustments. This is actually very common. The work you did brought you to a certain point and you may have made some remarkable changes. In order to get to the next level, additional adjustments are required. This is a new body you have compared to what you used to have. Its caloric needs, fitness level, and metabolic rate have all changed. Your new body needs a new approach. It won't be anything that is beyond your capabilities or exceptionally radical, just something a little more advanced than what worked for you previously. This is one of the reasons that I preach not doing more than is necessary initially. If you have been over-training and/or over-dieting, then you are stuck with very few options once your progress slows as it ultimately will on any program. By holding back initially, you now still have plenty of room to make changes.

Hidden Calories: Remembering that it is always easier to avoid calories than to burn them, it's best to look at possible nutritional changes first. If keeping your food log again didn't bring out any obvious red flags, it may be time to look at a few "hidden" culprits. Are you adding anything to your food or meals that might contain extra unwanted calories? A chicken breast, baked potato, and tossed green salad may seem like a nice "clean" meal. But if you are putting a high in sugar BBQ sauce on the chicken, butter and sour cream on the potato, and a high in fat or sugar dressing on your salad, your "clean meal" just turned into a nice little weight-gain meal. Of course this doesn't mean that you can't flavor or spice up your foods with seasonings. It just means that you must factor in anything that affects your caloric intake and consider it as a part of your diet. In the initial stages these hidden calories may not be as relevant because the other changes you make as far as food selection are more important. Now however, as you get further down the road, every little thing will weigh-in to a greater degree. Try switching to low-calorie dressings, sauces, and seasonings and utilizing products like "I Can't Believe it's not Butter" (an Elaine Goodlad staple). Most grocery departments have sections of products geared towards people who desire to be weight and health conscious. Also, there are many natural food stores which will give you an even greater opportunity to select and explore items that may fit well into your diet. The main point is that as you try to reach the next level, you have to start taking everything into account and make sure that you are not having anything negative to such a degree that it might hold you back.

Another thing to look at is your beverage consumption. Are you drinking a lot of calories without really considering them? Fruit juices are one of my favorite things and they can be quite healthy but they contain a lot of carbohydrates so you must be careful because it is quite easy for the calories to start adding up with a few glasses a day. If you are consuming any alcoholic beverages you should make sure to take this into account during your analysis of your nutrition program. Alcohol contains about 7 calories per gram plus the beverage may contain other carbohydrates as well. Try to consume fluids that will not add unwanted calories to your diet like Crystal Light, decaf iced tea, a limited amount of diet sodas, and of course, pure, clean water. Drinking adequate water, along with keeping the body properly hydrated will help you process and assimilate the foods you eat. It will help keep your metabolism working at peak efficiency and will also aid in combating hunger pangs by contributing to a feeling of fullness. Also, water is a natural diuretic and drinking plenty of water helps keep the body from holding excess water.

Another thing to look at is how you are actually preparing your foods. Baked, broiled, grilled, and even barbequed will always be preferable in terms of helping you get leaner than say, fried. Also try to avoid regularly consuming dishes where the necessary ingredients make it next to impossible for them to meet your diet parameters like lasagna. Leave foods like this as your occasional fun foods or cheat meal but really monitor and guard against them becoming a regular part of your diet.

Carbohydrate Manipulation: If you have determined that your diet is relatively clean and free from any hidden progress-slowing barriers, there are still a few "tricks" I have kept in reserve to help kick-start your progress again. First of all, always remember that you want to coax the body into change as opposed to trying to force it. The human body is always striving to maintain homeostasis or a proper balance. If you push it too hard in one direction, it will rebound in the other direction as it endeavors to again find balance. That's why eating more often causes you to burn more calories, restricting calories will cause you to store more calories, drinking lots of water will make you eliminate more water, not dinking as much water will cause you to hold water, etc. One of the reasons I wanted you to build up to eating 5-6 meals a day, aside from increasing your metabolic rate, is that it gives you a lot of meal possibilities in which you can manipulate your diet and coax your body into changing and becoming leaner. When you hit a sticking point or plateau, your body has become efficient at utilizing exactly how many calories you are giving it. So what you need to do is either give it a little less than it's going to burn or get it to burn more than it normally does. The most effective approach is to do both and there are a couple of steps that are involved.

Step 1: Add another complex carb meal for 2-3 days. The reason for doing this is that since your body is metabolizing everything fine we want to see if we can get it to metabolize a little more. One extra carb meal for 2-3 days will not add any appreciable amount of weight but it will put you in a better position to coax your body into a change.

Step 2: Switch all of you complex carb meals to slow digesting carbs. These are the carbohydrates that take longer for your body to digest and therefore require you to use more calories to complete the digestion process. This, along with that extra carb meal which is also a slow digesting carb should activate your metabolism just enough for our purposes.

Step 3: Pull the extra complex carb meal that you added, but stay with slow-digesting carbs. After 2-3 days of extra complex carbs, go back to the previous amount you were eating for a couple of days and see if you start losing.

Step 4: Replace a slow complex carb meal with fibrous carbs only. Now you are actually taking in fewer calories than you were, plus the calories you are consuming should take more energy to metabolize. This is the stage where most people will start to lose again. You've kick started your metabolism with a few days of extra food, then reduced your intake slightly and switched to a more energy demanding intake. You're not hungry, your metabolism is still racing along, and you're consuming fewer calories. Not much else for the body to do but lose weight. If it's still being stubborn go to Step 5.

Step 5: Remove a second complex carb meal replacing it with fibrous carbs. Up your protein and water intake if you'd like to help combat any hunger, but your food volume won't have changed too much so this probably won't be a problem. Continue this for three days and then add one complex carb meal, either slow or medium, to your diet.

This program works best if you are taking in at least three or four meals containing complex carbs (and remember-all of your meals should contain protein) originally because you will cycle up to five or six meals with complex carbs and then back down to one or two for a few days. The carbohydrate rotation takes 7-8 days to complete and in many cases will really jump start your metabolism. Of course it can be modified but always add at least one extra complex carb meal for a couple of days, change to slow digesting carbs, and then rotate down to at least one complex carb meal below normal. You can continue to implement this procedure, rotating up and down in complex carb containing meals and staying at each point for two-three days at a time based on how your body is responding. You shouldn't have to go lower than one complex carb meal even if it's a medium speed of digestion carb. Yes, there are advanced and extreme versions of this but don't go overboard and slow down your metabolism by doing this for too long or too often. Remember, your goal is to get lean on as many calories as possible, not as few. This is just a way to manipulate your diet and affect your metabolism to get you going again when/if you hit a plateau. Once you are losing again at a normal rate, rotate your intake back up to the highest point you can and still maintain that rate. This will probably be just slightly lower than the amount you were consuming before you hit your sticking point and you shouldn't have any trouble staying with it.

The only way this won't work for you is if you have already reduced your complex carb intake down to next to nothing and you don't have anywhere to go. You are basically at a point where you need to teach your body to be able to metabolize carbohydrates again by re-introducing them into your diet. Add an extra slow carb meal for 2-3 days, then add another one for 2-3 more days. Your weight will go up some because one part carbohydrate stores about three parts water (hence the name carbo-HYDRATE) so don't let this worry you. Next, remove the last slow carb meal you added, which should cause you to lose the weight you gained over the preceding few days and then you will actually be eating more than your were, with a metabolism that is hopefully on the comeback trail. Don't get confused by all these numbers and rotation schemes. The main thing to remember is to not reduce your complex carb intake to the point where you have nowhere else to go if you have more weight you wish to lose. If you do, you will be forced to temporarily halt your weight-loss efforts as you endeavor to jump start your metabolism.

You're stuck and nothing is working:

Breaking out with Training: As I stated before, nutrition is a bigger key to successful weight-loss than is training, but the combination of training and nutrition works better than either of them alone. If you find that you have hit a sticking point, there are also some things you can do in your workouts to break through to new progress. If you were at the beginning stages of exercise and fitness, it simply may be that you have graduated to another level that will require you to make a more concerted effort. Initially, any physical activity was enough to help you progress but now your body may have adapted and you are in better shape than before, thus needing to create a greater challenge for yourself. This is actually a good thing because it means you are becoming more fit and healthy. It is now up to you to modify your exercise program and make it more challenging and therefore, more productive. This may mean doing a more advanced form of training if you were previously a beginner, or it may simply mean doing more at your current level if you already are utilizing as advanced a form of training as you desire or have available. The bottom line is that you must create a greater physical challenge to receive a greater physical benefit.

Whether you are a beginner or quite advanced, there are a number of ways to increase your workout effectiveness. A common mistake that people make is assuming that more is better. Sometimes it is, sometimes it is not. The key is to do the things that will create the desired response by your body, both short-term and long-term. And there is a systematic way in which to do this that will be easy and effective.

Step 1: Make sure you are combining resistance training and cardio work in your overall program. If you are already doing this, great. But if you are only doing one and never do the other, this is the first change you need to make in order to effectively improve your physique. Also, don't forget the importance of a stretching/flexibility program, but for effective weight control, combining cardio and resistance training will give you the best possible results.

Step 2: If you already have a complete training program, try adding another day. This is one of the easiest and best ways to get you progressing again. Not only do you get the calorie burning benefit of another workout, you also get the post-workout metabolism boost as well. It doesn't have to be a monster workout that you add. It can just be an extra cardio day or an extra weight day or a combination if you like. Your ability to add an extra workout day will depend a lot on your schedule. If you are only working out three times a week, then I would strongly recommend going to that fourth day if you can. This is where the "lifestyle" part really kicks in. This is also why I didn't want you to start out doing more than was necessary. If you are already working out four days a week, yes you could add a fifth, but first check out the next step and make sure you are already meeting those parameters as there might be a better option for you. Your extra workout day can also be something apart from your normal exercise program. Maybe this could be the day to try that kickboxing or spinning class at the gym you've been hearing about. It could also be a good day to try out your skills in a sport you've wanted to take a crack at like soccer, volleyball, basketball, fitness walking, swimming, cycling, or even a fun run. It can be whatever you feel like doing as long as it gives you a workout that has additional fitness benefits. This is a great way to keep your fitness program both fun and productive.

Step 3: Bring your current workouts up to a level of greater intensity. In the same way that you took a step back and evaluated your diet to see if it was the best it could be, you can also take a look at your workout program to determine if it is still meeting your needs. The first step is to make sure you are training with the proper intensity. Over time your body has adapted and improved from the workouts you were doing. Those once challenging workouts may no longer be meeting your current fitness needs and therefore require adjustments. You can make them more difficult, and thus more productive, by increasing either the volume and/or the intensity of the workouts. Increasing the workout volume simply means doing more work, like adding another set to each exercise in your resistance training or increasing the length of your cardio sessions during your aerobic work. Intensity increase generally means working harder or at a higher level. Examples of this would be using heavier weights or imposing shorter rest periods during your resistance training, and going at a faster pace and/or higher level or elevation during your cardio work. The truth of the matter is that there is an almost infinite number of ways to increase both volume and intensity in your training as determined by a multitude of individual variables. It is impossible for me to accurately give you the exact details for your ideal workout because so many of you will be at so many different levels. Suffice it to say that eventually, your body will adapt to the lower levels of training and you may discover the need for your workouts to evolve as you get closer to your goals.

For those of you who have achieved a higher experience level, based upon what I know of your goal to get leaner and more fit, I can offer some basic parameters to consider that I have seen work quite effectively for many people. For resistance training: 3-4 workouts a week, 2-3 body parts a workout, 3 exercises per body part, 3-4 sets each exercise, 10-15 repetitions per set (select a weight that causes you to reach "form failure" somewhere in that range) with a 60-90 second rest period between sets is the general starting point I use for clients looking for maximum results. These parameters will have you using a weight that is not too light or heavy and working the muscles in a way that will develop them with maximum quality as opposed to maximum size or strength. Use longer rest periods and lower rep ranges if you would like to develop more size and strength.

For cardio, initially try to limit your workouts to no more than 30 minutes at a time and work up to four days a week. Increase the intensity of the cardio if you need it to be more challenging. While going for longer periods of time can be good with cardio training, a lot of people tend to pace themselves in order to go longer and longer and never really get the full benefit of this type of training. **By learning to work within a prescribed time period, you can increase the efficiency and effectiveness of your workouts.**

Once you have gotten all that you can from four cardio sessions a week at 30 minutes, then you can add a fifth session of 20-30 minutes on a different day. Better to do an extra workout than to keep going longer and longer on your other days. Once you've reached five days at 30 minutes, for some of you it may help to add 10 minutes to two of your 30 minute sessions but don't exceed 40 minutes at one time or else you will start burning more muscle than body fat (and begin to slow down your resting metabolic rate). Many people think that the way to get leaner is to keep adding more and more cardio but this is a dangerous trap. For most people, if you're not responding from doing four to five 30 minute sessions a week, it is not more cardio that you need but another look at your eating habits to get them back in line.

Step 4: Split your workouts to train more days. If you have been doing your resistance training and cardio training together, you may find it beneficial to separate the two, at least one day a week. By dividing your workouts up into either different times of day or different days entirely, you will have more energy for each workout session and you will have additional times and days at which you now expend calories and elevate your metabolism. An example of this would be to do your cardio in the morning and your resistance work in the evening. Another would be to not do any cardio on your most difficult resistance day, and do that cardio session with maybe an extra 10 minutes added on to it the following day (still not going over 40 minutes). The purpose of splitting your training is to be able to keep evolving your workout intensity to fit your body's needs and also create other opportunities to burn calories and boost your metabolism. Certainly don't go out and start training six days a week, twice a day. This is simply a way to take three workouts to four, four workouts to five, etc. in order to help you keep progressing and combat those nasty plateaus and sticking points. Once you've gotten to the point where your schedule is about as full as it can be, then you can up your cardio in terms of length if you still find that you need a greater challenge. At this point adding 10 minutes of cardio for two of your sessions will give you an extra 20 minutes a week. Slowly add time to additional sessions but remember, if you are doing more than five 30-40 minute cardio sessions a week and still not progressing, I would recommend you look in another direction to solve the problem.

You're still stuck and nothing works:

Breaking out with Nutrition: Ok, so you've re-evaluated your diet, tried carb rotation and manipulation, upped your training intensity and efficiency, and you say you're still stuck? Don't worry, I still have a couple of tricks/solutions up my sleeve. One of the reasons your progress has stopped could be that you are so close to your goal your body is just resisting losing any more fat because it perceives your fat stores as already being either too low or low enough. Congratulations if this is the case because you are almost there! It might be time for you to back off for a second and ask yourself if you know the difference between how lean you want to be and how lean you should be. Some body fat is normal, necessary, and healthy. You certainly don't want to go beyond what is ideal for your health. Simply by maintaining your weight at a certain point, you will look leaner over time as your skin continues to thin out and you gain back any lost muscle size and/or lose any excess subcutaneous water. Give yourself a little time and view yourself as objectively as possible. If you determine that you still need to continue getting leaner, there are a couple of good options left.

Option # 1: This option is for those of you who are down to the very last 4-6 pounds you need to lose and your body is being stubborn. Over the past few months you have restructured your metabolism, making it more active and hopefully you are still eating 5-6 meals a day. The thing to do now is simply eliminate a meal. If you have been eating 5 times a day, with a meal every 3 hours or so, now eat only 4 times a day with a meal every 4 hours. Going a little longer between meals with an active metabolism will cause your body to dip into its own energy reserves and you should start losing weight again. Yes, your body will eventually adjust metabolically and the weight-loss will stop, but it should continue long enough for you to lose those last few pounds you were trying to get rid of. This is a good strategy if you have an event a couple of weeks away and you are just trying to tighten up a bit. The two weeks gives you plenty of time to lose that last few pounds. So there you are, at your ideal target weight, eating 4 times a day, happy as a lark. But don't forget to go back up to your original meal count once the event is over. Remember the goal is to get lean on as many calories as possible and eat healthy all the time. You don't want to start slowing your metabolism back down again by depriving yourself over the long haul. By this point you should know your body pretty well and how it responds to a number of different variables so any adjustments you need to make won't be too difficult to figure out as you will already have all the tools and all of the experience. Pat yourself on the back for how well you've done and for how well you will continue to do!

Option #2: This option is for those of you who are completely stuck, nothing is working and you definitely have more than 4-6 pounds to lose. First of all, don't let yourself feel bad or become discouraged. You've simply been saddled with one of those troublesome metabolisms that makes everything more difficult than it should be through no fault of your own. You should still feel very proud of how hard you have been working and everything you have accomplished. And you should know without any doubt whatsoever that you will reach all of your goals. The thing you need to do now is very simple: you need to gain weight! Before you start thinking that I am crazy, hold on. Remember when I told you how fat-loss gets progressively harder as you get leaner? Remember also when I told you that the more weight you need to lose, the easier it is to do so? Also, I hope you recall what I said about the metabolism and how it needs to be coaxed and even tricked into responding as opposed to being forced. Well, this is the ultimate form of trickery and it works every time!

If you are doing everything right and nothing is working, you may have just reached a metabolic set point and you are experiencing diminishing returns for your efforts. Rather than go on some excessively radical exercise or starvation plan, you simply need to back off a bit, give yourself a break and then start anew. Take a week off from both your training and your weight-loss diet and just do what you feel, without any guilt. Eat some of your fun food favorites and engage in some enjoyable hobbies that maybe you had put on hold for a while. Yes, you will gain some weight, but not as much as you probably think. Besides, you are trying to gain weight, remember? Recall that the body is very over-reactive as it tries to maintain homeostasis. The more calories you eat, the more calories you burn. The more fats you eat, the more enzymes your body will produce to burn fat. Yes, there comes a point when this approach would lead to problems for you, but that point is not one week, trust me. The few pounds you gain will not be difficult to lose as you get back on your program but by then you should have picked up the metabolic momentum necessary to continue losing noticeably more than you gained. The body never stays the same. It is always changing in some way or another. Throughout the course of the day you are both gaining and losing weight, the one that you are doing to the greatest degree will determine your ultimate outcome. In this instance we are simply establishing and prolonging a weight-gain period for you to combat a resistive metabolism in order to take advantage of the rebound effect.

I remember a friend of mine who was as dedicated as anyone I ever met. When she was getting ready for competition no one could ever out work her. She would diet harder and harder and train more and more until everyone became amazed by her commitment. The problem was that the harder she seemed to work, the slower her progress became. She would get to the point where she was working out seven days a week, doing six days a week of weight training, six to seven days of cardio at 2-3 hours a day and consuming only around 900 calories daily. Unfortunately, the only thing she succeeded in doing was shutting down her metabolism. She never was able to get very lean on this program and when she started eating and training "normally" again, she would gain a lot of weight rapidly as her body rebounded from her excessive behavior. Once she gained back all to the weight she lost and then some, she would start the whole insane process all over again. Ultimately she was able to break the cycle by not starting off so intensely and following a program a lot closer to what I am recommending for you. The thing to remember is the rebound effect she experienced actually works both ways. The same way in which she stimulated her body to gain by losing, so can you stimulate your body to lose by gaining. This is a common practice among competitors who must peak for multiple competitions. Instead of impossibly trying to hold on to a certain level of conditioning, it's best just to back off the program for awhile and re-peak, getting even leaner than before. When all else fails, giving yourself that physical, mental, and emotional rest from your program will allow you to come back better and stronger and again be on your way to success.

CHAPTER 8

The Earth is not Flat!

It is sometimes difficult to accept a new idea or concept. As humans we are creatures of habit and develop various patterns and comfort zones. We watch the same things, go to the same places, wear the same style of clothes, listen to the same songs, sit in the same seats, eat the same foods, etc. as if we are trying to have some type of control over our lives. So when we hear something that is new to us we are often a bit slow to accept it.

Although much of the information I am presenting here is far from new, it may very well be new to a lot of readers simply because it is not what is currently being taught. With respect to weight loss, what we hear quite often is information referring to either trying to burn more calories or consume fewer calories, and if you have any type of weight management issues, that is where your answer lies. The problem is that this is an overly simplistic way to view weight loss and it operates on the assumption that the person in question is simply taking in too many calories and is not active enough. Sometimes this is true but very often it is not. In the many cases when this is not the issue, motivated and well intentioned people find themselves eating less and less and exercising more and more and experiencing great frustration as the success they seek to achieve never takes place. Once sufficiently frustrated, some people are almost wiling to try anything. Unfortunately many of them have been taken advantage of and led down the wrong path.

In all my seminars, personal training sessions, nutritional consultations and writings, the most difficult thing I've had to do has not been helping someone achieve success, it has been getting them to believe in and try the approach that I am advocating. We have been so conditioned to think, feel, and believe a certain way that it is hard for new ideas (even though they're really not that new) to be accepted and embraced. I have literally felt in some of the places where I presented seminars as if I was trying to convince people that the earth was not flat. They had a certain mentality that was supported by their peers and their fitness environment and even by the media. Add to this the number of times many of them had been promised, "This is the new, best, solve-all-your problems, answer-to-your-prayers diet!" and it's not hard to understand why they had their guards up.

What they couldn't see however is that the absolute easiest thing for me to do would have been to tell them something that they already believed and had heard. It would have given me instant credibility in their eyes and I would have received nothing but support. "Of course it's flat, we already knew that, but at least you know what you're talking about," I can almost hear them say. For me to come in and tell them something a little different must have meant that I had a good reason. And I did, I wanted to tell them the truth. I wanted to give them the best information possible that I felt would help them the most. I wanted to tell them how the body really worked, why many of them had not achieved success from the things they were doing and what the people who had been highly successful did as a matter of standard practice. I gave them what really worked, even if it may have been contrary to what they currently believed or were putting into practice.

I had girls/women who were taking 10-12-14-plus, 1-1 ½ hour long cardio classes a week on two-three meals a day. Many of them were stuck and not progressing. I told them that they needed to cut back on their cardio, up their meal frequency, increase their protein intake and add some weight training to their program to build and maintain muscle. I tried my best to teach them a better way. Although some listened, many more didn't. In my effort to teach I learned quite a bit. I discovered that it is not just enough to have better or even the best information. You have to be able to feed it to people in a way they would be willing to consume it so to speak. I couldn't just tell people what to do, I also had to help them understand why. For some, even this wasn't enough. I actually had to prove it to them. I brought in people I had worked with previously and people who followed the principles I was advocating for them to see and question and learn from and become inspired by. I found that it was a lot easier reaching new people through already successful ones. Nothing gets other women's attention quite like a sensational looking 40-year-old mother of two teenagers in a two-piece swimsuit, practicing her posing for her first figure competition. Being able to deliver the information through others became a way for me to reach more people.

Once getting people to try this "new" way became easier, I discovered that I still had one more big obstacle. While some people can make a few changes and immediately see positive results, for others it takes a while longer for good things to happen. In fact, for women who've been exercising extremely hard with a lot of cardio, little or no weight training, and an insufficient protein intake, their metabolisms could be shut down to such a degree that it will take weeks before they will start seeing the progress they want. In fact, for many of these women, because they have lost so much muscle tissue they will actually gain weight before their body is ready to start losing it again. Although the reasons for this are quite understandable, you can imaging how tough it is for them (and me) when they start on this "new" diet program and start gaining weight! All the doubts that I had worked so hard to erase came immediately back. It was compounded by the fact that by the time many of these women came to me for help they were almost desperate for progress. **"I've tried everything!"** was a common statement I heard. It had gotten to the point for some of them where they had attached a lot of their self esteem and sense of worth to their physical condition. They didn't dare miss one of those 10-12 classes a week. They couldn't imagine taking a break from their diet. They weighed themselves every single day, sometimes several times a day and their moods and emotions were attached to the raising or lowering of the numbers on the scale. It was starting to get unhealthy for some of them. That is not what fitness should be about.

Ironically the body has a way of letting us know this. If we are doing things incorrectly, either by working too hard or not hard enough, it will stop progressing the way it should. Just as a great number of people have not achieved their fitness goals due to a lack of commitment and effort, there is also a number of people who have not achieved success because of too great a commitment and too much effort. Remember, the body can only change and progress so fast and it prioritizes survival not appearance. If there is anything I have learned and can pass on it is this: **The body is in charge!**

If you happen to fall into the category of someone who has basically been trying too hard and have put your system into survival mode, it is very possible that you will gain some body weight when you first employ the principles I am advocating. You have probably lost a certain amount of muscle due to all the cardio and lack of adequate protein. Once you increase your protein intake and implement resistance training you will gain it back (as well as experience an increased metabolic rate). If your carb intake has been too low your muscle glycogen stores have been depleted. When you start consuming carbs again your muscles will store some of them, and since 1 part carbohydrates stores 3 parts water that will add a bit to the scale. Also, many over-trainers are simply a bit dehydrated much of the time and their body will rebound from this by temporarily storing more water than normal once they first began to take in an adequate amount of fluids.

All of the overtraining and under-nourishing has put your body in such a caloric deficit for so long that it has created an ideal condition for it to super compensate. In other words your body "feels' and "thinks" that you are in danger and will now try to protect against any further shortages by holding onto and storing whatever it has and whatever it is given. As un-ideal as this may seem, this is actually a good thing in that it is the first step in healing your metabolism. Your body is now getting proper nourishment and can begin to come out of survival mode. How long will this last and how much will you gain? It really depends on how severe the damage is and how long it has been going on. The longer you have put yourself through extreme diet and training approaches the longer it will take for your body to understand that it is no longer in danger and can safely start to work properly without risk of further assault.

The reason I am addressing this is that I want you to understand how critical it is to give yourself the amount of time necessary to start making progress. I have worked with women who became frustrated after only a few weeks of not seeing results (and possibly being 5-6 pounds heavier) and resorted back to their previous ways of doing things. Those women lost the 5-6 pounds they gained and then became stuck again (as they were originally) 15-20 pounds from where they really wanted to be. Others who were more patient eventually noticed (usually after 2-3 more weeks) that they were finally starting to change and at that point all limits were removed and they went on to reach their goals (and beyond!). The key ingredient is patience. Not all people will get an initial weight gain. And the ones who do the gaining will soon stop and as their metabolisms begin to pick up, their bodies will start getting leaner and lighter. This information I am giving you will work for you if you let it. Don't let 3-4 weeks of your body adjusting to change cause you to become frustrated to the point where you stop doing things they way that you should and rob yourself of 3-4 months (and possibly years) of good progress. Believe in the process and stay on course to your destination. You won't fall off the edge of the earth, I promise you.

CHAPTER 9

The Bodysport Diet: A Quick Review

If you want to look the best you can possibly look, there is a right way and a wrong way to do things. When I first started to introduce this information I was met with a lot of skepticism from people who were not familiar with it. Many of them had been training for quite some time and were very set in their ways. After convincing a few to try what I already knew to be tried and true methods based on how our body actually works more and more people started to come around. I used our competition website to illustrate the level of development that was possible with time. All the competitors and all the fitness models practiced methods very similar to what I was advocating. At first many people could not see how this related to them. But after watching some of their friends and associates put the information into practice and get results better than they ever had before, many began to see the light. "Tell me more about that Bodysport Diet," one of them asked me. I was only too happy to oblige. Here is an overview of the principles we have covered.

1. Establish a goal for yourself. What is it that you want to accomplish over the next several weeks or months? This can be a general goal like improving your eating and exercise habits, or more specific goals like losing a certain amount of inches or working out a certain number of times per week. Proceeding without some type of goal is like driving without a clear destination; you probably won't wind up where you most want to be. The key is to give yourself positive focus and direction.

2. Understand and accept the need for change if you want to make improvements. You cannot continue to do (or not do) the exact same things you have always done and expect a different or better result. The necessary changes may be quite small and should be easily manageable, but be prepared to have to implement something different to some degree.

3. Create a detailed and accurate food log. Write down everything you eat and drink along with the times you eat them for 5-7 days. This is to give you information about your current diet and to help you create an awareness of your own habits. Having this information will allow you to make the necessary changes to the appropriate degree. Without knowing what you are doing, you won't know what to change.

4. Look to eliminate the obvious obstacles first. These are the things that you know are not helping you, the "fun foods". This doesn't mean that you can never have them. It just means that you must make sure not to have them to the extent that they will keep you from progressing at the desired rate.

5. Stay out of starvation/survival mode. Remember, our body "thinks" in terms of survival first. If it's not getting what it feels it needs, the metabolism slows down and it starts conserving energy. At that point your body wants to hold on to everything it has (fat) and everything you feed it. It also wants to minimize energy output which it will do by reducing muscle since muscle burns calories when we are at rest. The last thing you want is to have your body trying to hold on to and store fat while simultaneously eliminating the muscle which keeps our metabolism active. The two big factors for keeping out of survival mode are as follows:

.

6. Regularly eat 5-6 meals a day. Ideally you want to progress to the point where you are eating at least 5 meals a day and approximately every 3-3 ½ hours. This is extremely important. By feeding ourselves regularly, we give the body the nutrients it needs to keep our metabolism active and keep it out of survival/starvation mode. Also, when we do go prolonged periods of time without eating, our blood sugar gets too low which can cause cravings and give us less control over making the right choices. Then, when we eat, our blood sugar elevates too rapidly and to such a great degree that we secrete insulin to get that excess sugar under control by converting it into stored fat. Eating frequently throughout the day helps stabilize the blood sugar and helps prevent this from occurring. If you are only eating 2-3 meals a day, work up to eating at least 5 by adding another meal every week or two.

7. Make sure to have protein with every scheduled meal. The difference between eating "five times" a day and "five meals" a day is that a meal has a set structure. Every single meal should have an adequate amount of protein. This will vary from person to person based on body weight, goals, etc., but generally speaking at least 20-25 grams of protein for women and 30-35 grams of protein for men should be consumed with *each and every meal*.

This is one of the biggest changes for most dieters and there are a few good reasons why this is so important. If you don't give your body protein regularly throughout the day, when it needs amino acids (the building blocks of protein) it will break down your muscle tissue to get them. This loss of lean mass makes your metabolism that much slower. Plus, if you eat meals that contain only carbohydrates, it has that previously mentioned effect on the blood sugar which also leads to more stored fat. Having protein each meal helps to stabilize the blood sugar level, build/maintain lean tissue (muscle), and also slows the digestion rate which causes you to expend more calories to process your food. For a great many dieters, especially women, the biggest reason for a lack of success is getting too little protein at each meal and throughout the day. Simply changing the protein/carb ratio in your diet, even without a reduction in calories, can have a noticeable and lasting effect on your long-term progress.

8. Have complex carbs with the first meal and fibrous carbs with the last meal. You should never completely eliminate carbohydrate foods from your diet. They contain too many quality nutrients like vitamins, minerals, anti-oxidants, fiber, water, etc. Plus, they are a great source of energy which is key for those of you who are working out as part of your fitness program. You simply need to have them when your body will most need them and use them. This means having an adequate amount of complex carbs with your first meal (remember every meal has a set amount of protein) to help "break your fast" and the lower-calorie fibrous carbs at your last meal when you will be less active. For your other meals, use your energy needs to help determine if you should consume complex carbs and how much you should have. Always ask yourself, "What will I be doing until my next meal?" At the times you will be more active, you will need to eat more complex carbs. At the times you will be less active, you would be better served eating a minimal amount of complex carbs or only fibrous carbs at that meal. This gives you more control over your diet and insures that you will have energy during the times of day that you need it, but are not taking in excess energy calories to be stored when you don't. This is a lot more effective than simply evenly dividing calories up throughout the day. Try it and you'll see.

9. Don't try to lose weight, try to lose fat or get leaner. A lot of people focus too much on simply changing the scale. This can be deceiving. You should focus on losing fat and getting leaner. You should also focus on building and/or maintaining muscle to keep your metabolism as active as possible. A good exercise program will go a long way towards making these things happen. Remember, the combination of exercise and diet will always be more effective than either of them alone. I talked extensively about the role of exercise and how to implement it earlier but generally speaking you need; cardio training for fat loss and aerobic conditioning, weight or resistance training for strength, muscle development and tone, and stretching for improved flexibility, recovery, and maximum functionality.

10. Think both long and short term. Pick a date or event approximately 3-4 months away as extra motivation to focus on as a target. Everyday as it gets closer it will keep you aware of trying to reach your goals. But for the immediate future, focus on the changes you need to make to get 5-7 pounds leaner. Remember, your body will only change so fast so all you need to do is make and/or continue the necessary changes and adjustments that keep you moving in the right direction. Imagine the "new look" you will have by the time that date arrives.

11. Believe in yourself. Believe in your ability to reach all of your goals and accomplish the things you want. There is no reason you won't be successful with time and effort. Enjoy the fact that you have started your journey and that you are now on your way!

BONUS CHAPTER

Principles of Nutrition for Athletes

One thing I have found is that frequently after someone successfully adopts a fitness lifestyle they progress to the point where they want to involve themselves in sports and competitions. While the principles of this book are pretty universal and adaptable, I thought you might like to take a look at nutrition from an athlete's point of view. Toward that end I have included for you a piece I wrote on the role of nutrition as it relates to athletes or anyone involved in maximizing physical performance:

The biggest favor athletes can do for themselves is to embrace the value of nutrition and the overall importance of diet to their success. Nutrition by definition is the consumption, digestion, and assimilation of foods and other nutrients for conversion into structural compounds (skin, muscle, hair, etc.) and functional processes (growth, energy, metabolic maintenance, etc.). The value of nutrition ranges from basic survival to optimal health and culminates for the athlete into maximum performance. Nutrients can be either essential (those which cannot be produced by the body), or non-essential (those which can be manufactured from other nutrients). These nutrients are derived from food and are divided into macronutrients (water, protein carbohydrates, and fats) and micronutrients (vitamins, minerals, and trace elements). It is the regular consumption of food nutrients that makes up a diet. Contrary to popular belief, a diet is not something that someone goes on or off. It is simply the sum total of all foods and beverages consumed by an individual. It can be either good or bad depending upon the needs of the individual and the items selected for consumption. The periodic adjustment of the diet is what allows an individual to reach specific goals. By understanding the cause and effect relationship of nutrition and using proper dietary manipulations, an athlete can maximize their potential to succeed.

Obviously, we all need basic nutrients to survive. Just the fact that you are reading this proves that those needs are being met. There has also been enough literature to make people aware of the need for a minimal amount of particular nutrients in order to maintain health and remain free of disease. In fact, that's what the RDA (Recommended Daily Allowance) refers to, the minimum amount necessary. But for an athlete to truly excel, they must concern themselves with getting the optimal amount of the nutrients necessary for good health and maximum performance in relation to the increased demands that will be placed upon the body. You must be able to give your body what it needs, when it needs it, to promote health, energy, recovery, and ideal body composition. And the first step to this is understanding the basic elements of food and how they effect you.

Macronutrients are the food elements required daily in quantities determined by weight, usually ounces or grams, which ultimately provide the energy necessary to maintain body functions during rest and physical activity. Macronutrients also provide the materials necessary for structural growth, maintenance, and repair. Calories, the measurable heat energy of food that can be either utilized or stored, are provided by the macronutrients. Protein and carbohydrates each contain approximately 4 kcal per gram with fat containing 9 kcal per gram and alcohol 7 kcal per gram. (kcal=kilocalories but is most commonly referred to as just calories)

Micronutrients are the vitamins, minerals, trace elements, and bio molecules required by the body in small amounts, usually measured in milligrams and micrograms. They act as cofactors in making other bio molecules and function as enzymes, electrolytes, catalyst, and have some structural roles. They do not provide a significant amount of calories but in some cases can contribute greatly to disease prevention and the maintenance of optimal health.

The seven elements of food; protein, carbohydrates, fats, vitamins, minerals, water, and trace elements, all combine to make up the foundational components of nutrition. Each has it own definitive purpose and role:

Protein-Long chains of amino acids that have a number of structural functions. Protein comprises 80% of the dry weight of muscle and 90% of the dry weight of blood. It is the macronutrient most responsible for the growth and repair of tissue and can be derived from both plant and animal sources. An athlete must be conscious of consuming protein periodically throughout the day. Ingested protein is broken down by the body into its building blocks, the amino acids, before it can then be assimilated and utilized for innumerable functions. The proper balance between protein intake versus protein breakdown is of vital importance.

Carbohydrates-High energy containing macronutrients that are composed of carbon, hydrogen and oxygen in chemical substances that include sugars, starches, glycogen, dextrose, and cellulose. Carbohydrates contain the body's main source of the raw materials for energy and are classified as either simple or complex. The body stores carbohydrates in the muscles and liver as glycogen. Since excess carbohydrate intake beyond energy and recovery needs can lead to fat storage, carbohydrate manipulation is one of the keys to controlling body composition. Different types of carbohydrates have varying effects on the blood sugar level of the body which can also be a major factor in manipulating body composition.

Fats-As the most concentrated source of energy in the diet, fats contain more than twice the energy of carbs or protein. Fats are made up of saturated fatty acids which come primarily from animal sources and are solid at room temperature, and unsaturated fatty acids which come primarily from vegetables, seeds, and nuts, and are usually liquid. Fats, also known as lipids, by definition are soluble in organic solvents but not in water. Fats are essential to health and also have many important structural functions. Generally speaking, humans consume too much of the wrong types of fats and not enough of the good fats. The different types of lipids include; triglycerides, fatty acids, essential fatty acids, Omega 3 fatty acids, Gamma Linolenic Acid, Medium Chain Triglycerides, Phospholipids, lecithin, and cholesterol. Triglycerides make up about 98% of all the fats in the diet.

Vitamins-These are organic food substances found in both plants and animals that are essential in small amounts for numerous metabolic functions, energy production, and normal good health. Vitamins are generally classified as either fat soluble or water soluble and can be derived from foods and additional supplementation. The deficiencies of certain vitamins can lead to severe medical conditions and an adequate amount is considered beneficial for optimal athletic performance.

Minerals-These are inorganic compounds that are essential nutrients required by the body in very small amounts. They are important in many structural and metabolic roles and make up 4-6% of the body. They are categorized as macro minerals, trace elements and electrolytes and can be as important as vitamins to overall health and athletic performance. Dietary surveys have determined that most athletes' diets are deficient in one or more minerals.

Water-As the most vital of all nutrients, water can make up as much as 70% of a persons body mass. Water aids in the digestion, transportation, and assimilation of all other nutrients. It also aids in heat stabilization as it absorbs considerable heat with only small changes in temperature. It is vitally important for all athletes to maintain proper water balance and remain properly hydrated at all times. The body derives water from consuming liquids, ingesting foods, particularly fruits and vegetables, and metabolic water produced when food molecules become metabolized for energy.

The Three Primary Functions of Nutrition for Athletes

Hydration- It is generally recommended in sports nutrition that an athlete consumes at least 1 pint of fluids 2 hours before activity. This will give enough time for optimum absorption and the elimination of excess fluids. To combat dehydration during training or competition, athletes must always remember that their bodies may need fluids before they actually experience the sensation of thirst. Enough fluids must be consumed to replace that which is lost due to perspiration and respiration. This will also be affected by environmental conditions such as heat and humidity. Consuming 6-8 fl. oz. every 15-20 minutes is a good starting point. Post workout or competition, athletes must be conscious to re-hydrate themselves properly. Fluids should be consumed at a rate of 1 pint for every pound of lost body weight. Athletes should re-gain all lost water-weight before their next workout.

Energy-The foods and beverages that an athlete consumes can have a direct effect on their training and performance. The energy that an athlete has available for training and competition is determined by their general nutritional habits as well as their specific pre-workout or competition practices. Athletes who consistently eat high quality foods geared towards fueling their bodies with proper nutrients will greatly improve their ability to maximize performance. The quantity, quality, and timing of meals will all be factors in developing proper pre-event nutrition practices.

Recovery-The physical demands that are made upon the body by an athlete causes the loss of critical nutrients and it is imperative to the athlete to replace these nutrients through proper nutrition. Athletes must always be conscious of their post-workout nutritional needs and look to fuel the body as quickly and as efficiently as possible in order to insure maximum recovery and energy replacement. The ability to store carbohydrates or glycogen is maximized right after a workout and proper storage of this energy nutrient will greatly determine the rate at which an athlete will be physically prepared for their next practice or event.

Having a general knowledge and understanding of the basic components of nutrition and its importance to athletic success will serve as a foundation to further learning and dietary practices. This will allow each athlete to determine and implement the specific, individual nutritional programs needed to maximize their training and their performance.

Conclusion: A New Beginning

If I have learned anything about fitness over the past 30 years, it is that the more you involve yourself in it, the more it becomes a part of you. The goal of losing weight or getting leaner is one shared by millions. It can either become a journey of terrible frustration or tremendous triumph. A lot of this has to do with getting the proper information and not being led astray. When the initial desire for improvement is combined with the satisfaction of success, tremendous drive and momentum can be built up. A passion for health and life can soon develop that carries over into all things. The great thing is that this can happen long before all of our goals are reached. I have personally learned much in my ongoing quest for self improvement and neither the journey nor my enlightenment has yet to reach an end. As you continue to discover your own personal fitness lifestyle, don't forget to applaud yourself for the distance you have come and enjoy the excitement of the accomplishments still ahead. Don't let anyone or anything discourage or stop you from being what and who you want to be. Continue to find inspiration in everything, both success and setback. Your desire for success has caused you to increase your knowledge so that with time and effort you will accomplish great things. Let this be a great start to an even greater future. You don't deserve anything less.

Appendix and Friends:

The following appendix contains both the **Carbohydrate Rate of Digestion** sheet and **Nutritional Value of Foods** sheets. Use these to help with your food selection and meal planning as you create your diet. There are a number of references sources where you can find more food listings and nutritional information but this should give you a good start on some of the most common items. These are the exact same lists that I give to the people I coach. I recently came across an online source for nutritional food values at www.nutritiondata.com. On this site, you can simply type in the name of a food and get all kinds of useful information, a wonderful tool to have.

For those of you who haven't grown tired of me, I still plan to be around. Right now I am involved in the re-working of our Bodysport website with my business partner Terry Goodlad. The new format will be a weekly fitness magazine geared not only towards women interested in competing in the sports of Figure and Fitness, but will cover all aspects of training, nutrition, motivation and living a positive, healthy lifestyle. We will have a writing staff and advisory board made up of many of the top people in the fitness industry who will be contributing regularly. Bodysport contains a lot of wonderful and useful information for anyone who is serious about fitness. www.Bodysport.com.

I will also soon have my own fitness information and motivation site. It will contain tons of information to help you on your fitness journey as well as highlight the accomplishments of some truly motivational people who are living the fitness lifestyle. www.performafit.com (coming soon)

I am very fortunate to have many friends in the fitness industry. Check out the Bodysport.com link's page for a full list but here are some that I think will be of particular interest to you;

Elaine Goodlad- IFBB Figure Pro and top fitness model (one of my favorite people ever!) www.elainefit.com

David Sandler- President of **StrenghtPro**, a Sports Performance Enhancement Company, David is a world leader in the fields of strength and conditioning and fitness. www.strengthpro.com

Tanya Merryman- Fitness America National Champion, IFBB Fitness and Figure Pro, personal trainer and top group exercise instructor- A long time friend, Tanya is group exercise director for the new UFC gyms. www.tanyam.com

Nancy Georges- Top fitness professional and coach. Nancy is a great motivator and role model. One of the industry's most respected people. www.nancygeorges.com

Carla Sanchez- IFBB Fitness Pro, top trainer, coach, and head of The Performance Ready Team. www.carlasanchez.com

Ana Tigre- Fitness fashion designer of cutting edge workout and urban wear. Ana is also a top National level figure competitor. www.yourbelezabrazil.com and www.sweetrevengeclothing.com

Bodysport TV- Inspiring and motivational fitness video site where you can watch and learn and even upload your own fitness related videos. www.bodysporttv.com

Bodysport Fitness Center- Owned by our friend Mel Fabros, a private training studio in Las Vegas, NV. www.bodysportvegas.com

Nutrient Food Values

Protein: 3.5 ounces trimmed of visible fat

	P	C	F
Skinless Chicken Breast	31g	0g	4g
Skinless Turkey Breast	30g	0g	1g
Top Round	36g	0g	4g
Top Sirloin	30g	0g	6g
Salmon	27g	0g	7g
Halibut	27g	0g	3g
Lean Ground Beef	28g	0g	16g
Shrimp	21g	0g	1g
Shark	21g	0g	5g
Deli Roast Beef	28g	7g	4g
Deli Ham	21g	2g	6g
Pork Tenderloin	28g	0g	5g
Canned Tuna	25g	0g	1g
Red Snapper	26g	0g	2g
Egg Whites (6)	24g	2g	0g

Eggs Whole (6)	36g	6g	30g
Plain non-fat Yogurt 8oz	13g	17g	tr
1% Cottage Cheese 1c	28g	6g	2g
Milk non-fat 1c	8g	12g	tr
Veggie Burger 1 patty	14g	11g	2g
Veggie Chik-N 1 patty	14g	11g	2g
Garden Burger 1 patty	10g	8g	2g

Complex Carbs: 1 cup cooked unless indicated

	P	C	F
Oatmeal	6g	25g	2g
Plain Bagel, 1	7g	38g	1g
White Rice	4g	44g	tr
Brown Rice	5g	45g	2g
Macaroni	7g	40g	1g
Spaghetti	7g	40g	1g
Whole Wheat Bread (1 slice)	3g	13g	1g
Corn Tortilla, 1	2g	12g	1g
English Muffin, 1	5g	25g	1g

	P	C	F
Black Beans, ½ c	8g	20g	1g
Lentils, ½ c	9g	20g	tr
Kidney Beans ½ c	8g	20g	tr
Potato, 1	5g	51g	tr
Sweet Potato, 1	2g	28g	tr
Tomato, 1lg	2g	8g	tr
Corn ½ c	3g	21g	1g
Avocado, ¼	1g	3g	8g

Fruits:

	P	C	F
Strawberries 1c	1g	11g	tr
Apple, 1	tr	21g	tr
Orange, 1	1g	16g	tr
Grapefruit, ½	tr	9g	0
Banana, 1	1g	28g	tr
Peach, 1	tr	11g	tr
Pineapple, 1c	tr	19g	tr
Pear, 1	tr	25g	tr
Raisins, ¼ c	1g	29g	tr

Apricots, 3	1g	12g	tr
Blueberries, 1c	1g	20g	tr
Plum, 1	tr	9g	tr
Nectarine, 1	1g	16g	tr
Kiwi, 1	tr	11g	tr
Watermelon 1c	1g	12g	0
Raspberries	1g	15g	1g

Nuts:

	P	C	F
Peanut Butter 2tbsp	8g	6g	16g
Almonds 1oz	6g	5g	15g
Walnuts 1oz	7g	3g	16g
Peanuts 1oz	7g	6g	14g
Cashews 1oz	4g	9g	13g
Pecans 1oz	3g	4g	21g
Flaxseed oil 3tbsp	5g	11g	10g

Fibrous Carbs:

	P	C	F
Broccoli, 1c raw	2g	4g	tr
Spinach, 1c	1g	1g	tr
Zucchini, ½ c	tr	4g	tr
Corn ½ c	3g	21g	1g
Romaine lettuce 1c	1g	1g	1g
Mushrooms, 1c	2g	3g	tr
Salsa, ½ c	1g	6g	tr
Cucumber, 1c	1g	3g	tr
Carrot, 1	1g	7g	tr
Onion, 1c	2g	14g	tr
Collard Greens, 1c	tr	3g	tr
Bell Pepper 1c	1g	10g	tr
Green Beans, ½ c	1g	5g	tr
Asparagus, 4 spears	1g	3g	tr

Carbohydrate Digestion Rate

Slow Digesting Carbs:

Apples
Beans
Brown Rice
Yams
Rye Bread
Yogurt
All Fibrous Carbs (except corn and carrots)

Medium Digesting Carbs:

Oatmeal
Corn
Fruits
Red Potatoes
Peas
White Rice
Pastas
Buckwheat noodles and pancakes

Fast Digesting Carbs:

Cold Cereals
Cream of rice and wheat
Simple carb drinks
White bread
Honey
Instant Potatoes
Carrots
Glucose

©2009 Kevin Myles

6499269R0

Made in the USA
Lexington, KY
25 August 2010